What you need to know
ABOUT
Vitamins, Minerals, & Supplements

BY GAYLE SKOWRONSKI & BETH ROYBAL

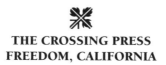

THE CROSSING PRESS
FREEDOM, CALIFORNIA

Copyright © 1998 by Gayle Skowronski & Beth Roybal
Cover design by Victoria May
Interior design by Magnolia Studio
Printed in the U.S.A.

No part of this publication may be reproduced or transmitted in any form or by any means, electric or mechanical, including photocopy, recording, or any information storage and retrieval system now known or to be invented, without permission in writing from the publisher, except by a reviewer who wishes to quote brief passages in connection with a review written for inclusion in a magazine, newspaper, or broadcast. Contact The Crossing Press, Inc., P.O Box 1048, Freedom, CA 95019.

All rights reserved.

For information on bulk purchases or group discounts for this and other Crossing Press titles, please contact our Special Sales Manager at 800-777-1048.

Visit our Web site on the Internet: www.crossingpress.com

Disclaimer:
The information contained in this book is not intended as a substitute for consulting with your physician or other health care provider. Any attempt to diagnose and treat an illness should be done under the direction of a health care professional. The publisher does not advocate the use of any particular health care protocol, but believes that the information in this book should be available to the public. The publisher and author are not responsible for any adverse effects or consequences resulting from the use of any of the suggestions, preparations, or procedures discussed in this book.

Library of Congress Cataloging-in-Publication Data

Skowronski, Gayle.
    Vitamins, minerals & supplements / by Gayle Skowronski & Beth Roybal.
        p. cm. -- (Vital information series)
    Includes index.
    ISBN 0-89594-935-0 (pbk.)
    1. Vitamins in human nutrition. 2. Minerals in human nutrition. 3. Dietary supplements. I. Roybal, Beth Ann Petro. II. Title. III. Series.
QP771.S57   1998
613.2'8--dc21   98-26909
                                                                 CIP

Contents

INTRODUCTION 5

CHAPTER 1: WHY TAKE A SUPPLEMENT? 7
The ABCs of Nutrition 7
Supplementation: An Ongoing Debate 19
Considering a Nutritional Supplement 24
The Bottom Line—It's Up to You 28

CHAPTER 2: VITAMINS 29
Vitamins and Your Health 29
Fat- and Water-soluble Vitamins 30
Antioxidants 31
Vitamin A and Beta-carotene 33
Vitamin B_1 (Thiamin) 36
Vitamin B_2 (Riboflavin) 38
Vitamin B_3 (Niacin or Nicotinic Acid) 39
Vitamin B_5 (Pantothenic Acid) 41
Vitamin B_6 (Pyridoxine) 41
Vitamin B_{12} 42
Vitamin B_{15} (Pangamic Acid) 44
Biotin 44
Folic Acid (Folate or Folicin) 44
Lecithin (Phosphatidylcholine or PC) 48
Para-amino Benzoic Acid (PABA) 48
Vitamin C 48
Vitamin D 52
Vitamin E (Alpha-tocopherol) 55
Vitamin K 57
Vitamin Q 59

CHAPTER 3: MINERALS 60
The Role of Minerals in Your Body 60

Mineral Deficiencies 62
Mineral Toxicity 63
When to Supplement 63
Boron 64
Calcium 65
Chromium 68
Copper 69
Fluoride 71
Iodine 72
Iron 74
Magnesium 76
Manganese 79
Molybdenum 80
Phosphorus 82
Potassium 83
Selenium 85
Sodium 87
Zinc 89

CHAPTER 4: OTHER NONHERBAL SUPPLEMENTS 92
Who Needs Nonherbal Supplements, Anyway? 92
Supplement Safety 93
Common Forms of Supplements 94
Categories of Supplements 95
Enzymes 96
Amino Acids 99
Essential Amino Acids 100
Nonessential Amino Acids 108
Essential Fatty Acids 116
Other Supplements 118

**CHAPTER 5: CROSS REFERENCE OF NUTRIENTS
            BY HEALTH CONDITION 123**

REFERENCES 134

INDEX 135

Introduction

Vitamins. Minerals. Nonherbal supplements. Just what are they? What roles do they play inside the body? Who needs them? How should they be used? How much is enough? Can too much hurt me?

If you have questions like these, then this is the book for you. This book provides general information about the role of supplements in nutrition and how to choose supplements wisely. The book also gives details for specific common nutritional supplements, including the following descriptions:

▲ The role of the nutrient in the body

▲ What happens when your body experiences a deficit of the nutrient

▲ The amount of the nutrient needed daily to maintain good health

▲ When additional amounts might be appropriate

▲ Cautions to keep in mind when using the supplement

Keep in mind that there are also thousands of herbal, or more appropriately, "botanical" supplements available. While many vitamins, minerals, and supplements contain substances that come from plant sources (often called phytonutrients), herbal preparations are not covered in this book.

But before reading further, you should be aware that there is a fair amount of controversy about supplements, both theoretical (whether there is ever any reason to use supplements when eating a well-balanced diet, for example) as well as practical (such as skepticism about the health benefits attributed to specific supplements). These ongoing debates—with opponents often holding extreme and uncompromising positions—can make it difficult for you to decide whether or not to use a given supplement. What we attempt to do in this book is to present the information as completely and objectively as possible. We have no particular point of view to protect: We are neither doctors, nor nutritionists, nor health practitioners. We are simply writers who enjoy presenting complex health information to people in a way that they can really use. It's entirely up to you to decide how to incorporate this information into your quest for better health.

There is one position we do hold to strongly, however: Nutritional supplements should not replace a healthy lifestyle. You know what we mean—all those things your doctor, your significant other, or that little voice in your head keep reminding you about:

▲ Eating a well-balanced diet

▲ Getting regular, moderate exercise

▲ Keeping stress under control

▲ Avoiding abusive substances and risky behaviors

We encourage you to view nutritional supplements exactly as the word implies—as a possibly useful addition to your overall plan for enjoying a healthy, fulfilling life. We'll talk more about that later.

But now, it's time to choose how you wish to use this book. If you want to simply look up specific nutrients, then go directly to the appropriate chapter:

▲ Chapter 2: Vitamins

▲ Chapter 3: Minerals

▲ Chapter 4: Nonherbal Supplements

If you don't know which category the nutrient belongs to, then check the table of contents or index first. If you're looking for which vitamins, minerals, and supplements are useful in treating specific health conditions, go to Chapter 5.

If, on the other hand, you want a little more background about nutritional supplements, turn the page to Chapter 1 and read on.

CHAPTER 1

Why Take a Supplement?

Is there ever a good reason to use a vitamin, mineral, or nonherbal supplement? Some reputable nutrition experts say, "Yes, of course," while others just as knowledgeable say, "No way." Despite the controversy, at least a quarter of us just go ahead and take nutritional supplements anyway.

There is no definitive answer to the dilemma of whether or not to use a nutritional supplement, but you can consider the evidence and come to your own conclusions. This chapter should help. It begins by reviewing the various perspectives on dietary supplements, pro and con. We also discuss reasons why you might consider supplementation, as well as general cautions to keep in mind when selecting and using supplements.

THE ABCs OF NUTRITION

Before launching into the debate about whether supplementation is necessary or desirable, it may help to take a few minutes to review some basics about nutrition and its role in health. We'll start by looking at what you ate for lunch.

COMPONENTS OF FOOD

Whether you munched on a juicy cheeseburger with all the fixings, a Lean Cuisine fresh out of the microwave, a few spoonfuls of natural vanilla-flavored yogurt, or a salad packed with sprouts and veggies, the food you ate was broken down by your digestive system into several components. One group of these is called macronutrients, which provide your body with energy, measured by calories. Macronutrients include the following:

▲ **Carbohydrates** form the largest category of macronutrients. Carbohydrates come from plant sources and range from complex to simple. As they are digested, carbohydrates are broken into increasingly simpler forms of sugar. Eventually, they are stored in the liver and other cells throughout the body as glucose. Many foods containing complex carbohydrates also contain fiber, although fiber is not actually carbohydrate and is not digested. Fiber comes in two forms: soluble and insoluble. Soluble fiber absorbs water during the digestive process, making stools soft. Insoluble fiber does not absorb water. It provides the bulk which keeps food moving through your digestive system.

▲ **Fat** is also used by the body for energy. Fat breaks down less readily than carbohydrates. Once it is broken down, it is stored in cells throughout the body.

▲ **Proteins** are made up of various combinations of amino acids. Protein comes from both animal and plant sources. The liver can break apart protein into its acids and recombine them as needed. The amino acids that make up proteins are often available in supplemental forms and will be described in more detail in Chapter 4.

In addition to macronutrients, food is also made up of micronutrients, which you need in smaller quantities. Micronutrients do not break down to provide energy. Rather, they serve as catalysts, helping the body use macronutrients for energy. Micronutrients also perform many other functions in the body. Micronutrients include the following:

▲ **Vitamins** enable the body to release stored energy and to perform all sorts of other functions. Their roles will be discussed in more detail in Chapter 2.

▲ **Minerals** aid many functions of the body, such as keeping the body's electrical system in balance. They also help form cell walls. The function of various minerals will be described in Chapter 3.

- **Other micronutrients** include a variety of chemicals that aid body processes in other ways, such as enzymes to aid digestion. Many of these nutrients are available in supplemental form and will be discussed further in Chapter 4.

The food you ate for lunch contains varying amounts of these macro- and micronutrients. The cheeseburger, for example, would be filled with protein and fat, with decent doses of certain vitamins and minerals, while the salad would have less protein and fat, but more fiber and carbohydrates and high amounts of certain types of vitamins and minerals. As that bite of food slides down your throat and esophagus and drops into your stomach, strong acids begin the process of breaking down the food into its nutrient components. As digesting food passes through the stomach and intestines, the nutrients pass through the intestinal walls and are circulated to the appropriate parts of the body. Most of the nutrients pass through the liver first, which has the ability to break them down into even smaller components, a process called metabolism, and recombine them into new forms more easily used by the body. The liver also serves as a storage site for many nutrients, until the body needs them for a particular purpose or at a particular location.

DIETARY GUIDELINES

In order to ensure an adequate amount of the various nutrients, several dietary principles come into play. You may be most familiar with the US Department of Agriculture's Food Guide Pyramid. It serves as a quick visual reference for making wise daily food choices.

But more recently, many experts have backed off making such directive pronouncements about the numbers of fruit servings or carbohydrates needed to ensure adequate nutrition. Instead, nutritionists are preaching these basic principles:

- *Strive for variety.* Nutritional deficits occur in many otherwise normal, healthy people simply because they've grown accustomed to eating the same few foods over and over again.

▲ *Balance eating and activity to maintain or lose weight.* Getting regular exercise is almost as important as eating a balanced diet.

▲ *Choose foods low in fat.*

▲ *Enjoy all foods*—but don't overdo it.

Following these guidelines permits more latitude in selecting food based on your individual preferences.

Whether you follow the pyramid, these guiding principles, or some other scheme (in Canada, the Food Rainbow reigns as the official message on what to eat, for example), the goal is the same—to make sure you get enough of the nutrients needed to maintain a healthy body. But how much is enough?

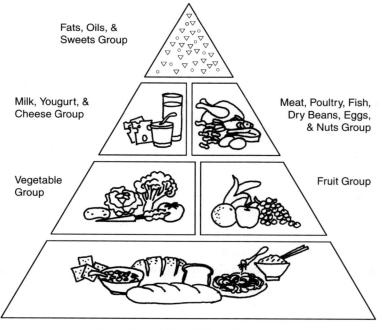

The Food Guide Pyramid

RECOMMENDED DAILY ALLOWANCES (RDA)

The National Institute of Medicine (**NIM**) branch of the US National Academy of Science (**NAS**) is the body responsible for determining the optimal levels of nutrients needed daily to maintain health. Since 1941, these levels have been reflected in the Recommended Dietary Allowances (**RDA**). You've most likely run into these numbers on the nutrition information labels found on most food products in the US. On these labels, the RDAs of relevant nutrients are included, as well as the percentage of RDA contained in a single serving of the product. The term used on the label is Daily Value (**DV**). Because the RDA is such a widely accepted standard, in this book we will refer to it extensively when discussing appropriate levels of nutrients.

Nutrition Facts
Serving Size 1/2 cup (56 g)
Servings Per Container 13

Amount Per Serving
Calories 210   Calories from Fat 45

	% Daily Value*
Total Fat 5 g	8%
Saturated Fat 0.5g	4%
Sodium 25mg	1%
Total Carbohydrate 35g	12%
Dietary Fiber 5g	18%
Sugars 9g	
Protein 7g	
Calcium 4% •	Iron 10%

Not a significant source of Cholesterol, Vitamin A and Vitamin C.
*Percent Daily Values are based on a 2,000 calorie diet.

Nutrition Facts from a Granola Product

You may also begin to see the term **RDI** (Reference Daily Intake) used. It is the same as RDA, but is now the USDA's preferred term.

You will also begin to see RDAs or RDIs on the backs of all nutritional supplement containers. There, too, the phrase Daily Value (**DV**) is used.

PERCENT DAILY VALUE FOR ADULTS AND
CHILDREN OVER 4 YEARS OF AGE

Vitamin A	5,000 I.U.	100%
Vitamin B-1	1.5 mg	100%
Vitamin B-2	1.7 mg	100%
Vitamin B6	1.0 mg	50%
Vitamin B12	3 mcg	50%
Vitamin C	50 mg	83%
Vitamin D	400 I.U.	100%
Vitamin E	10 I.U.	33%
Folic Acid	100 mcg	25%
Niacin	20 mg	100%
Calcium	125 mg	12.5%
Copper	1 mg	50%
Iodine	150 mcg	100%
Iron	5 mg	27.8%

*Supplement Facts from a Multivitamin/
Multimineral Supplement*

The RDAs you usually see in these two places reflect current consensus on healthy levels of various nutrients for a normal, healthy adult. In actuality, there are many different RDAs for any given nutrient, based on age, weight, sex, and special circumstances such as pregnancy and breastfeeding.

RECOMMENDED DIETARY ALLOWANCES
FOR INFANTS AND CHILDREN

NUTRIENT	INFANTS		CHILDREN		
	0–6 MOS (13 LBS)	6 MOS–1 YR (20 LBS)	1–3 YRS (29 LBS)	4–6 YRS (44 LBS)	7–10 YRS (52 LBS)
Energy (calories)	650	850	1300	1800	2000
Protein (grams)	13	14	16	24	28
Vitamin A (mcg of beta-carotene)	375	375	400	500	700
Vitamin D (mcg)	7.5	10	10	10	10
Vitamin E (mg of alpha-tocopherol)	3	4	6	7	7
Vitamin K (mcg)	5	10	15	20	30
Vitamin C (mg)	30	35	40	45	45
Thiamin (Vitamin B) (mg)	0.3	0.4	0.7	0.9	1.0
Riboflavin (mg)	0.4	0.5	0.8	1.1	1.2
Niacin (mg)	5	6	9	12	13
Vitamin B6 (mg)	0.3	0.6	1.0	1.1	1.4
Folate (mcg)	25	35	50	75	100
Vitamin B12 (mcg)	0.3	0.5	0.7	1.0	1.4
Calcium (mg)	400	600	800	800	800
Phosphorus (mg)	300	500	800	800	800
Magnesium (mg)	40	60	80	120	170
Iron (mg)	6	10	10	10	10
Zinc (mg)	5	5	10	10	10
Iodine (mcg)	40	50	70	90	120
Selenium (mcg)	10	15	20	20	30

RECOMMENDED DIETARY ALLOWANCES FOR MEN

NUTRIENT	CHILDREN		ADULTS		
	11-14 YRS (99 LBS)	15-18 YRS (145 LBS)	19-24 YRS (160 LBS)	25-50 YRS (174 LBS)	51+ YRS (170 LBS)
Energy (calories)	2500	3000	2900	2900	2300
Protein (grams)	45	59	58	63	63
Vitamin A (mcg of beta-carotene)	1000	1000	1000	1000	1000
Vitamin D (mcg)	10	10	10	5	5
Vitamin E (mg of alpha-tocopherol)	10	10	10	10	10
Vitamin K mcg)	45	65	70	80	80
Vitamin C (mg)	50	60	60	60	60
Thiamin (Vitamin B) (mg)	1.3	1.5	1.5	1.5	1.2
Riboflavin (mg)	1.5	1.8	1.7	1.7	1.4
Niacin (mg)	17	20	19	19	15
Vitamin B6 (mg)	1.7	2.0	2.0	2.0	2.0
Folate (mcg)	150	200	200	200	200
Vitamin B12 (mcg)	2.0	2.0	2.0	2.0	2.0
Calcium (mg)	1200	1200	1200	800	800
Phosphorus (mg)	1200	1200	1200	800	800
Magnesium (mg)	270	400	350	350	350
Iron (mg)	12	12	10	10	10
Zinc (mg)	15	15	15	15	15
Iodine (mcg)	150	150	150	150	150
Selenium (mcg)	40	50	70	70	70

RECOMMENDED DIETARY ALLOWANCES FOR WOMEN

NUTRIENT	CHILDREN		ADULTS		
	11-14 YRS (101 LBS)	15-18 YRS (120 LBS)	19-24 YRS (128 LBS)	25-50 YRS (138 LBS)	51+ YRS (143 LBS)
Energy (calories)	2200	2200	2200	2200	1900
Protein (grams)	46	44	46	50	50
Vitamin A (mcg of beta-carotene)	800	800	800	800	800
Vitamin D (mcg)	10	10	10	5	5
Vitamin E (mg of alpha-tocopherol)	8	8	8	8	8
Vitamin K (mcg)	45	55	60	65	65
Vitamin C	50	60	60	60	60
Thiamin (Vitamin B) (mg)	1.1	1.1	1.1	1.1	1.0
Riboflavin (mg)	1.3	1.3	1.3	1.3	1.2
Niacin (mg)	15	15	15	15	13
Vitamin B6 (mg)	1.4	1.5	1.6	1.6	1.6
Folate (mcg)	150	180	180	180	180
Vitamin B12 (mcg)	2.0	2.0	2.0	2.0	2.0
Calcium (mg)	1200	1200	1200	800	800
Phosphorus (mg)	1200	1200	1200	800	800
Magnesium (mg)	280	300	280	280	280
Iron (mg)	15	15	15	15	10
Zinc (mg)	12	12	12	12	12
Iodine (mcg)	150	150	150	150	150
Selenium (mcg)	45	50	55	55	55

RECOMMENDED DIETARY ALLOWANCES FOR PREGNANT AND BREASTFEEDING WOMEN

NUTRIENT	PREGNANT WOMEN	BREASTFEEDING WOMEN (FIRST 6 MOS)	BREASTFEEDING WOMEN (SECOND 6 MOS)
Energy (calories)	+300	+500	+500
Protein (grams)	60	65	62
Vitamin A (mcg of beta-carotene)	800	1300	1200
Vitamin D (mcg)	10	10	10
Vitamin E (mg of alpha-tocopherol)	10	12	11
Vitamin K (mcg)	65	65	65
Vitamin C (mg)	70	95	90
Thiamin (Vitamin B) (mg)	1.5	1.6	1.6
Riboflavin (mg)	1.6	1.8	1.7
Niacin (mg)	17	20	20
Vitamin B6 (mg)	2.2	2.1	2.1
Folate (mcg)	400	280	260
Vitamin B12 (mcg)	2.2	2.6	2.6
Calcium (mg)	1200	1200	1200
Phosphorus (mg)	1200	1200	1200
Magnesium (mg)	320	355	340
Iron (mg)	30	15	15
Zinc (mg)	15	19	16
Iodine (mcg)	175	200	200
Selenium (mcg)	65	75	75

Even though a range of RDAs exist for most vitamins and many minerals, the opposite is also true. For some very important nutrients such as chromium, no RDAs have yet been established. This is the case for many minerals and most other nutritional elements.

DIETARY REFERENCE INTAKES (DRIS)

Because of the growing realization within the scientific community that so little is understood about optimal levels of nutrients, the RDA has become part of a larger description of the nutritional picture. This larger category is called the Dietary Reference Intake (**DRI**). It is used by both the US and Canada and incorporates the following four levels of nutrient intake:

- ▲ *RDA:* The minimum daily intake needed to prevent deficiency

- ▲ *Adequate Intake (**AI**):* Estimated amounts of nutrients needed to maintain health, used when there is not enough scientific evidence to determine a particular RDA. AI is based on experimental or observational data. For example, AIs are being set up for infants based on the average nutritional intake of breastfed babies.

- ▲ *Estimated Average Requirement (**EAR**):* The amount of nutrient needed to maintain health for half the people in a given group. This number is used by nutrition experts to determine RDAs. Since the primary use of the EAR is to help in establishing or revising RDAs, it's unlikely you will run into this nutritional measurement.

- ▲ *Tolerable Upper Intake Level (**TUIL**):* The maximum level of a nutrient, above which adverse effects may occur. The NIM is quick to point out, though, that in most cases there is no proven benefit for taking nutrients at levels above the RDA and below the TUIL.

DRIs represent a major shift in thinking about nutrients. Use of the RDAs alone kept the focus on preventing nutritional deficiencies. Nutrients for which no RDAs existed were often ignored. Incorporating other measures of nutrients recognizes that it may be desirable to have an intake of nutrients in addition to the minimal levels established by the RDAs. In fact, an increasing number of studies point to the benefits of large doses of nutrients in treating several medical conditions. Adopting the concept of DRIs essentially acknowledges that increasing the intake of certain nutrients can have healthful or even medicinal benefits.

The DRIs are a breakthrough in how the scientific community views nutrition. However, at this point DRIs have been established for only a few nutrients: calcium, phosphorus, magnesium, vitamin D, and fluoride. Over the next several years, DRIs will be developed for other nutrients as well, as funding becomes available (these studies rely on grants from other governmental agencies and private manufacturers).

PUTTING RDA AND DRI TO WORK FOR YOU

How can RDA and DRI help you? They give you baselines from which to develop a nutritional plan of action. Because percentages of RDAs are listed on most food products and are available for other foods (such as fruits and vegetables), you can estimate the amount that you eat of most vitamins and minerals. If you have major deficiencies, this should show up immediately and you can take steps to correct them through changes in diet or by supplementation. DRIs serve as a cautionary upper limit, above which toxicity can easily occur. If you find a need to supplement beyond the RDAs, the DRIs can help prevent severe side effects, or even death. For your reference, RDAs and DRIs will be incorporated into the descriptions of nutritional supplements in Chapters 2 and 3.

A NOTE ABOUT ALL THOSE MEASUREMENTS

You may see several abbreviations after the numbers indicating nutrient levels. Here's a quick description of what those abbreviations mean:

▲ *mg: Milligram*

▲ *mcg: Microgram, one tenth of a milligram*

▲ *IU: International unit, a term that represents agreed-upon standards of measurement for a particular nutrient. Unlike mg and mcg, IU is not a constant figure. For example, 5000 IU of beta-carotene (vitamin A) is the equivalent of 5000 mcg or 5 mg of vitamin A. On the other hand, 200 IU of vitamin D is equivalent to 20 mcg or 0.2 mg of vitamin D. Wherever possible, we will give the mcg or mg equivalent when referring to IU.*

INTERNATIONAL DIETARY GUIDELINES

The World Health Organization (**WHO**) of the United Nations is in the process of formulating worldwide standards for dietary supplements. Some concern has arisen that these guidelines would be overly restrictive in comparison to guidelines already in place in the US. The US Food and Drug Administration (**FDA**) states it will not adopt any guidelines that impinge on the right of the US to regulate its own dietary supplement market.

SUPPLEMENTATION: AN ONGOING DEBATE

For years, medical doctors, dietitians, and most other traditional Western health care practitioners have maintained that nutritional supplements are almost always unnecessary. Theoretically, the argument makes sense: You should be able to get all your nutritive needs through the foods you eat. But reality may be otherwise. Many factors could lead to developing a nutritional deficit that needs supplementation:

- ▲ Increasing age
- ▲ Special circumstances such as being pregnant, breast-feeding, or undergoing a treatment that depletes a particular nutrient
- ▲ Inability to eat a normal diet
- ▲ Prolonged stress
- ▲ Exposure to environmental pollutants and toxins

In addition, there may be legitimate reasons to take a nutritional supplement above and beyond the amounts available through diet alone. Using supplementation might be appropriate for:

- ▲ Treating or alleviating symptoms of certain health conditions
- ▲ Preventing some types of health problems
- ▲ Enhancing your overall health and well-being

Let's take a closer look at these factors and how supplementation might be appropriate in these cases.

INCREASING AGE

Nutritional supplements may help you age "healthfully." The tendency to develop some nutritional deficits as you grow older is well documented. For instance, older people often lack enough of certain B vitamins. In most cases, these deficits are probably due to the body's growing inability to absorb nutrients as you get older. In addition, your body may have an increasingly difficult time processing or using the nutrients that are absorbed. Furthermore, there is growing recognition that older people may need higher levels of certain nutrients such as calcium than younger adults.

All of these factors may require that you increase your intake of some nutrients at a time when you may not be able to eat as much or as wide a variety of foods as you once did. Supplementation may be entirely appropriate for healthy aging.

SPECIAL CIRCUMSTANCES

Many special circumstances exist for which most health experts would agree that nutritional supplements are desirable. We'll describe several of these cases here.

Pregnancy is one condition for which there is almost universal agreement that a vitamin–mineral supplement should be taken daily. The justification is that adequate baseline levels of nutrients are critical to the development of the baby, while the risk of overdosing is very low. In fact, any woman who is considering becoming pregnant is encouraged to begin taking prenatal vitamins. Doctors even write prescriptions for prenatal vitamins, so that if you have prescription coverage through health insurance, the cost to you can be lower than if you buy them over-the-counter.

Breastfeeding mothers also need a higher level of nutrients— even higher than for pregnant women. After all, you're providing all or most of your newborn's nutrition for the first year, while at the same time continuing to supply your own nutritional needs. Most health care providers recommend that you continue taking prenatal vitamins as long as you breastfeed.

Treatments for cancer and other health conditions can often deplete certain nutrients. If you are undergoing chemotherapy, kidney dialysis, or any other treatment, check with your health care provider to see if you would benefit from supplements.

Smokers may have deficits of certain nutrients, such as vitamin C. Of course, the best solution is to quit, but in the meanwhile supplementation might be called for.

Drinkers of excessive amounts of alcohol also have nutritional deficits. Alcohol decreases the absorption and use of some nutrients. Also, heavy drinkers may not be eating enough.

INABILITY TO EAT A NORMAL DIET

You may be unable to eat a normal diet for many reasons:

- ▲ You may have a temporary illness, have an ongoing medical condition, or be recovering from surgery and find it difficult to eat enough to meet your nutritional needs.
- ▲ Certain critical foods simply may not "agree" with you, perhaps due to digestive disorders, gallbladder problems, or severe food allergies.
- ▲ You may be on a very low calorie diet for weight loss.
- ▲ You may be a strict vegetarian.

In all these cases, you may have a nutritional deficit.

PROLONGED STRESS OR EXPOSURE TO TOXINS

Stress, pollutants, and toxins can deplete your body of vital nutrients. This may occur even if you are "healthy" and meet the RDAs for nutrients through your diet.

TREATING OR ALLEVIATING SYMPTOMS OF CERTAIN HEALTH CONDITIONS

From vitamin A for improving eyesight to zinc as an antidote for impotence, people have looked to dietary supplements to provide cures and symptom relief that are unavailable from traditional medications. Anecdotal evidence and some more formal scientific studies indicate that people with a range of health conditions may benefit from the use of dietary supplements. Such evidence exists for rheumatoid and osteoarthritis, hepatitis, high blood pressure, high cholesterol, and many other diseases and conditions.

Unfortunately, in most cases little "hard" evidence for the role of supplementation exists. By hard evidence, we mean formal studies in which supplementation was monitored for one group of people and compared to people who had no supplementation. This type of testing is done all the time in new drug development. However, it is costly, complex, and time-consuming. Most research of this nature is sponsored by the company developing the product. Most manufacturers of nutritional supplements don't have the resources to conduct such thorough investigations. This picture is changing as small studies by many researchers on the use of various supplements accumulate. In addition, many pharmaceutical companies are gaining interest in nutritional supplements, rather than viewing them as threats to traditional pharmaceuticals. They will likely be funding studies as they purchase companies that manufacture supplements or add supplements to their product lines. However, there will probably be gray areas in proving the benefits of nutritional supplements for any given health condition, since it is almost impossible to control all the other factors (such as diet or medications) that could have affected the results.

In the meanwhile, individual reports of success in using various nutritional supplements are slowly accumulating. These findings are probably legitimate; however, they don't provide firm, broad guidelines for use of nutritional supplements. This places the burden of choice about whether to use a supplement squarely on your shoulders. Supplements are also used when treatment for a health condition, such as chemotherapy or another medication, depletes vital nutrients. See Chapter 5 for a list of health conditions with references to the nutrients linked with each condition.

PREVENTING SOME TYPES OF HEALTH PROBLEMS

Much as supplements may be useful in treating some health problems, they may also prevent certain health problems from occurring in the first place. Again, the evidence is fragmented. But the accumulation of studies over time is pointing to the role of certain dietary nutrients in preventing a variety of cancers, cataracts, high blood pressure, and other health problems. Again, since the evidence is not overwhelming in all cases, it is up to you to decide if nutritional supplements are appropriate in your circumstances.

ENHANCING YOUR OVERALL HEALTH AND WELL-BEING

But what if you're generally healthy and get adequate nutrition through your diet? Is there any reason for you to consider using nutritional supplements? Most traditional health care practitioners, such as your family doctor, would probably say an emphatic "No!" But others—such as the sellers of nutritional supplements—would disagree. Although there is the least amount of cold, hard scientific data to support such contentions, many users of nutritional supplements testify to how these supplements benefited them, even though they were suffering from no obvious health problem. What are some of these claims and how might they be true?

Nutritional supplements have been suggested for many reasons besides curing disease. Here are just a few:

▲ Enhancing athletic ability
▲ Improving sexual performance
▲ Sharpening memory, concentration, and other cognitive skills
▲ Providing more energy
▲ Calming frayed nerves
▲ Encouraging more restful sleep
▲ Maintaining or losing weight
▲ Improving a general sense of well-being

Are these claims all in the supplement users' heads? Perhaps. But there are many reasons that nutritional supplements could work to accomplish some of these effects. First, an individual may be suffering from a nutritional deficiency or health condition and not even know it. The supplement may simply be helping to return the user to an optimal state of health. Furthermore, if there is some evidence that dietary supplements can prevent certain health problems, it seems reasonable that they can also go beyond prevention to enhancement. These arguments are all theoretical, of course. But combined with the anecdotal reports of many supplement users, it forms at least a basis for deciding whether a nutritional supplement may be worth trying.

CONSIDERING A NUTRITIONAL SUPPLEMENT

If you have decided that it is appropriate for you to take a dietary supplement, then do so wisely. Don't just rush off to your nearest health food store and purchase the first supplement you see. Like any other product you buy, it's worth taking a few minutes to do your homework. Here are some areas to consider.

UNDERSTAND THE RISKS

The US Food and Drug Administration (**FDA**) only loosely regulates the dietary supplement market, partly because of budgetary constraints and partly because of legislation that was passed by Congress in 1994 that limits the FDA's role in regulating dietary supplements. They step in only if there has been a serious complaint about a particular product, as they did with L-tryptophan a few years ago when a defective batch caused illness in many people and several deaths. If there is evidence that a product causes problems, the FDA will issue advisories and, if necessary, take action. And when funds permit, the FDA will occasionally test products already on the store shelves. However, the FDA relies on the manufacturer to ensure the quality of the product. You should also keep in mind that the FDA has no jurisdiction over advertising claims—that is handled by the Federal Trade Commission (**FTC**).

As of 1997, the FDA has guidelines for makers of supplements to follow in labeling their products. These are similar to the FDA guidelines for labels that list nutrition facts for food products. Supplement labels should include the following:

- ▲ Identification of the product as a dietary supplement.
- ▲ A Supplement Facts panel, including a description of the "serving" size, information on the basic fourteen nutrients if present, and information for other nutrients that are present.
- ▲ A list of dietary ingredients that have no RDAs.
- ▲ The identity of each dietary ingredient.
- ▲ The part of the plant used, if the supplement contains botanical ingredients.

Under these guidelines, the term "high potency" can be used only when the amount of the nutrient exceeds 100 percent of the RDA. The term "antioxidant" can be used when the nutrient has been scientifically shown to have antioxidant properties (see the description of antioxidants in Chapter 2).

These new guidelines may seem rather basic; however, it is the first time any attempt has been made to standardize and require specific information on supplement labeling. While these guidelines provide some help for the consumer, there is still no guarantee that the supplement you buy is, in FDA lingo, "safe and effective." Chances are that the product is okay to use, but it's up to you to proceed with caution.

ASK FOR ADVICE

Direct any questions you have about a supplement to someone who is qualified to answer them. Of course, this advice is easier to say than to implement. You may be wondering just who is qualified to give such advice. Try some of these health professionals:

- ▲ Start with your primary care provider. Although many physicians know very little about dietary supplements, some have made an extra effort to learn more about them, especially if they have themselves had a positive experience with a dietary supplement. Furthermore, your physician, physician's assistant, or nurse practitioner may be able to refer you to someone who is more knowledgeable.

- ▲ A nutritionist (usually a credentialed professional with a master's degree) may be able to help. Some nutritionists have a conservative approach toward dietary supplements (that is, they believe they should rarely be used), while others have specialized in the area of supplemental nutrition, especially in relation to athletic performance or chronic health conditions.

- ▲ Someone with a background in biochemistry may at least be able to help you evaluate whether claims about a given supplement make sense.

▲ Contact the manufacturer's marketing department and ask for documentation of any product claims (specific citations from published studies, not their own publications).

In addition, the staff at stores that sell nutritional supplements are usually knowledgeable about their products and their uses.

KNOW YOUR SOURCE

Believe it or not, the most expensive product may not be the best. And what is the "best" product may depend on your own needs. When purchasing a nutritional supplement, ask yourself these questions:

▲ Is the source of the product reputable? It may be hard to judge this, but if a company has been in business several years, its products are probably okay.

▲ Where should I purchase the product? Traditionally, nutritional supplements have been carried primarily by stores that specialize in supplements or health food. However, many pharmacies now also carry a surprisingly wide range of dietary supplements. You may get more comprehensive advice from the traditional outlets, but you probably can't beat a drug store's price, especially if the store carries generic (non-branded) or store-labeled products.

▲ Does the supplement contain ingredients I don't want? Usually the supplement bottle will list ingredients and include the source of certain nutrients (such as thymic preparations from calves). Check the labeling carefully if you have any known food allergies. Occasionally ingredients such as whey or gluten are used. Sugar, salt, and other flavor enhancers may be added. And if you're a strict vegetarian, watch for products that use gelatin capsules from animal sources. Some newer vegetable-based capsules are available through a few companies, or buy a tablet, powder, or liquid form instead.

▲ Should I buy only "natural" products? Theoretically, synthetic and natural vitamins and minerals are chemically the same. Synthetic versions are usually cheaper to produce, and therefore less expensive to you. However, you may want to consider supplements claiming to be all natural if that is important to you. Also, the all-natural versions may contain other elements, known or unknown, which could be either helpful (such as a chemical that aids absorption) or harmful (such as contaminants).

MAKE THE MOST OF YOUR PURCHASE

Supplements aren't cheap. Make the most of your purchase by following these tips:

▲ Check the label for an expiration date. If the product has expired, it may have lost potency.

▲ Store supplements in a cool, dark location to preserve maximum potency. While you're at it, make sure the supplements are securely stored to prevent poisoning of children.

CHOOSE THE BEST COMBINATION

If you want to take a supplement that contains more than one nutrient, read labels carefully. Make sure the RDAs used on the label match the RDAs for your age and sex (see the charts earlier in this chapter). Some multisupplements are formulated for people with special needs, such as stress relief, cancer risk reduction, or digestion aid. Talk to your health care provider or pharmacist for advice.

AVOID EXCESS

Just because a little does you some good, doesn't mean a lot will do you even better. Sometimes "megadoses" can be helpful or therapeutic. But unless you are working with a qualified health professional who can monitor your use, it's best to err on the side of caution. For many vitamins and minerals, even a slight overdose can be toxic (poisonous to your body) or deadly. For others, taking too much is simply a waste of money—your body excretes the excess through your urine. And some nutrients when taken in too great of doses can inhibit the absorption of other nutrients. All good reasons not to overdo it—and to find out ahead of time the symptoms of toxicity for the supplement you are taking.

REPORT ANY PROBLEMS

Because the regulation of dietary supplements relies so heavily on the "honor system," it's important that you make your voice known if you have any problems with a supplement. Contact the manufacturer or, if you are unable to do so, the place where you purchased the supplement. You can also report adverse affects to the FDA at 1-800-FDA-1088 or via the FDA website at www.fda.gov/medwatch. If you prefer, your health care provider can also make a report, ensuring your confidentiality. Any complaints about product advertising should be directed to the FTC.

THE BOTTOM LINE—IT'S UP TO YOU

With a better understanding of the role of dietary supplements in nutrition, when supplementation might be appropriate, and how to choose supplements wisely, you now have the basic information you need to help you decide if you should try a nutritional supplement. The following chapters give you more details about specific supplemental nutrients.

CHAPTER 2

Vitamins

Carbon, oxygen, hydrogen, and nitrogen. These four chemicals combine in various groupings to form the different vitamins. Even though their makeup is similar, the effects of the different vitamins in the body are wide-ranging. First we'll take a look at this connection between vitamins, your body, and your health. Then we'll describe characteristics of fat-soluble vitamins, water-soluble vitamins, and antioxidant vitamins. Following that, you'll find information about each vitamin, including its role in the body, RDAs, sources of the vitamin, and considerations for supplementation.

The vitamins described here are available as single supplements, or you may find them in various amounts in multivitamin/multimineral supplements.

VITAMINS AND YOUR HEALTH

Vitamins don't give you energy directly—although most vitamins help release stored energy from the carbohydrates, protein, and fats you eat. In addition to helping release energy, vitamins fill many other critical roles in your body:

- ▲ Starting or speeding up chemical reactions within your cells (**catalysts**)
- ▲ Aiding the digestive process
- ▲ Helping your body resist infection
- ▲ Helping your body grow
- ▲ Keeping you mentally alert

Your body keeps a certain level of each vitamin in constant circulation in the blood, so that the vitamins are readily available to perform their functions when needed.

Your body cannot make most vitamins, so you need to get them in other ways, usually through the food you eat. There may be certain circumstances when you can't get enough of a particular vitamin through food or your need of the vitamin may be unusually high. In these cases, supplementation may be appropriate. This is especially true if you're over age 65. For older people, taking a multivitamin supplement may help your immune system to function better, preventing and fighting off infections more readily.

FAT- AND WATER-SOLUBLE VITAMINS

With one exception, vitamins fall into two groups: fat-soluble and water-soluble. The difference between the two matters for more than just the biochemist studying these micronutrients. Whether the vitamin is soluble in water or fat affects how it is stored in your body—and whether overdoses are toxic. Let's take a look at each type of vitamin.

WATER-SOLUBLE VITAMINS

The B vitamins (except vitamin B_{12}) and vitamin C dissolve in water. This means that your body cannot store them and that you need to have a constant supply of these vitamins. If you take more of these vitamins than your body can use, they are simply excreted out through your urine.

FAT-SOLUBLE VITAMINS

Vitamins A, D, E, and K dissolve in fat, not in water. Extra stores of these vitamins remain in your cells. This means that you don't need to have a steady supply of the fat-soluble vitamins. It also means that if you take too much of them over a period of time, toxic levels can build up, sometimes quickly. This is especially true for vitamins A and D.

THE EXCEPTION

Vitamin B_{12} is the lone exception. Rather than being flushed out through urine or stored in fat cells, B_{12} is stored in the liver. Like the fat-soluble vitamins, this means that you don't need a constant flow of the vitamin through your diet. But if levels of B_{12} accumulate, your liver can be damaged.

ANTIOXIDANTS

Antioxidants—especially vitamin E—have been pitched as the cure for almost anything. But what are they? And why are they so important? To answer these questions, let's take a look at how your body operates at the level of the cells.

CELLS CREATE FREE RADICALS

As the millions of cells in your body perform their normal tasks, they give off "exhaust"—called free radicals. Just like the exhaust from a car pollutes the environment, free radicals are toxic to the body. In fact, free radicals can also come from environmental pollution outside your body, such as car exhaust, cigarette smoke, or other chemicals floating through the air that you breathe in.

A free radical is a molecule that is lacking its full charge. It roams the body looking for extra charges from other sources. Once it finds this extra charge—let's say from a healthy cell in your blood, for example—the free radical steals the charge, leaving a damaged cell behind. This process is called oxidation.

The damage caused depends on where it occurs in the body and whether or not the free radicals are able to overwhelm your body's response to them. Take these examples:

- ▲ In the blood vessels, oxidation can cause a few "bad" LDL cholesterol cells to become damaged and stick to vessel walls. If nothing reverses the damage, damaged cells build up, clogging your blood vessels. Artery disease and even heart attacks can result.
- ▲ In the skin, oxidation causes benign wrinkles, undesirable age spots, or deadly skin cancers.
- ▲ Free radicals and the oxidation process can cause other types of cancers, as well.
- ▲ In the eyes, free radicals and oxidation may be the cause of cataracts.

What's to stop these marauders from taking over and destroying your body? That's where antioxidants come into play.

ANTIOXIDANTS DISABLE FREE RADICALS

Antioxidants are substances that carry extra charges. Simply put, they lend their extra charges to free radicals, preventing them from wreaking damage. At this point in time, it is believed that three vitamins serve as antioxidants in your body:

- ▲ Beta-carotene
- ▲ Vitamin C
- ▲ Vitamin E

Each antioxidant seems to work in different ways and in different areas of the body to prevent damage caused by free radicals. In general, these antioxidants seem to lower the damage associated with heart and artery problems, eye problems, and many types of cancer. Vitamin antioxidants don't seem to have a role in preventing breast cancer, however. In addition, some studies show that under certain circumstances antioxidants may be associated with or even cause health problems. One example is a link between smokers, beta-carotene, and lung cancer. Yet another complication to the antioxidant story is that no one is sure which dosage levels of which antioxidants would be most effective and whether it is more effective to eat foods high in these antioxidants or to take supplements.

IMPLICATIONS FOR YOUR HEALTH

Put all of this together, and what should you make of antioxidants? It's likely that eventually they will be proven to prevent or limit certain health problems. In the meanwhile, it certainly doesn't hurt to make sure you are getting the RDA for each antioxidant. For some people, it may make sense to supplement at even higher levels, especially if you're at risk for heart disease, cancer, or cataracts. For the rest of us, supplementing with antioxidants has no proven benefit, but probably involves little risk as long as you don't take too much of these potent vitamins. And it's likely that benefits of antioxidant therapy in generally well people will become better understood and documented in the years ahead.

> ## A NOTE ABOUT VITAMIN RDAs
>
> *Although the RDAs are developed by the National Institute of Medicine division of the US National Academy of Science, US government agencies are involved in the RDAs as well, including the Food and Drug Administration and the US Department of Agriculture. Each has adjusted the RDAs somewhat to reflect current thought, since the National Institute of Medicine's process for reevaluating the RDAs will not be completed for several years. This means that it is difficult to find consistent information about RDAs. In this section on vitamins, the National Institute of Medicine's RDAs are shown in the chart, with exceptions noted in the text below each chart.*

VITAMIN A AND BETA-CAROTENE

Sorting through the differences between vitamin A and beta-carotene can be confusing. Simply put, beta-carotene is a substance found in many foods. It is a member of a group of substances called carotenoids, including lutein and lycopene. As a group, carotenoids present researchers with exciting possibilities in improving our health. There is even some thought about establishing a RDA for carotenoids in general, separate from the vitamin A RDA.

But back to beta-carotene: Once you eat beta-carotene, the body converts it into a form it can use—vitamin A. Vitamin A itself is also available as an additive to some foods and in supplemental form, which your body uses directly. When considering adding vitamin A to your diet, you should know whether you are adding beta-carotene or vitamin A itself. Most supplements with vitamin A, for example, are really beta-carotene. In fact, the RDA for vitamin A is actually for beta-carotene, not for vitamin A.

VITAMIN A, BETA-CAROTENE, AND OTHER CAROTENOIDS' ROLE IN YOUR BODY

Your body doesn't use beta-carotene as it is, but converts it into vitamin A. The process begins as stomach acids encounter beta-carotene. In fact, low levels of stomach acid may lead to a deficiency in beta-carotene. This is most likely to occur in several groups of people:

▲ Almost one-third of adults over age 60, who may have lost their ability to generate enough stomach acids (this condition is called atrophic gastritis or hypochlorhydria)

▲ People with ulcers caused by the Helicobacter pilorii bacteria

▲ Others with digestive disorders that limit the production of stomach acid

▲ People taking certain medications that block the production of stomach acids

Researchers believe, but have not yet proven, that eating sour (**acidic**) foods may help increase the absorption of beta-carotene. Once absorbed and converted into vitamin A, some of it is circulated in the blood, some is stored in fat cells throughout the body, and the rest is stored in the liver. If you need to find out how much vitamin A is in your body, a liver biopsy is currently the best way to obtain this information, though blood tests are under development.

The antioxidant properties of beta-carotene, other carotenoids, and vitamin A have been linked to several health benefits:

▲ Preventing many types of cancer

▲ Preventing cataracts

▲ Preventing cholesterol buildup in your blood vessels (study results on the role of beta-carotene and cardiovascular disease have been mixed), and thus reducing risk for artery problems, heart attacks, and strokes

▲ Preventing some types of thyroid problems

In general, beta-carotene may have the effect of boosting the immune system, especially in the elderly. This effect was observed only with beta-carotene supplementation and not seen with the supplementation of vitamin A. Beta-carotene and similar carotenoid substances (**lutein** and **lycopene**) may also prevent colds and flu. Lycopene may also reduce skin damage caused by ultraviolet (**UV**) light.

RDA FOR VITAMIN A (BETA-CAROTENE)

The RDAs for vitamin A are really RDAs for beta-carotene. RDAs for other carotenoids have not been established.

RECOMMENDED DIETARY ALLOWANCES
FOR VITAMIN A (MCG OF BETA-CAROTENE)

AGE	WEIGHT	RDA
Infants 0–6 mos	(13 lbs)	375
Infants 6 mos–1 year	(20 lbs)	375
Children 1–3 years	(29 lbs)	400
Children 4–6 years	(44 lbs)	500
Children 7–10 years	(52 lbs)	700
Men 11 years and older		1000
Women 11 years and older		800
Pregnant Women		800
Breastfeeding Women (first 6 months)		1300
Breastfeeding Women (second 6 months)		1200

SOURCES OF BETA-CAROTENE AND VITAMIN A

Beta-carotene is found in many plants, usually dark green and deep yellow in color. These include the following:

▲ Broccoli

▲ Cantaloupe

▲ Carrots

▲ Sweet potatoes

▲ Winter squash

Other carotenoids are found in kale, tomatoes, pink grapefruit, and other red, orange, and yellow fruits and vegetables. "Preformed" vitamin A is found in animal products and is often added to cereals.

SUPPLEMENTS

No one has established strict guidelines for additional supplementation or whether supplementation should be with beta-carotene or vitamin A. Several studies have used 50 mg of beta-carotene given every other day.

The American College of Obstetrics and Gynecology recommends that pregnant women not take more than 5000 IU of vitamin A (beta-carotene) each day.

The other carotenoids, lutein and lycopene, are not currently available in supplement form.

CAUTIONS

As a fat-soluble vitamin, beta-carotene or vitamin A can become toxic since excess amounts are stored in the body, especially in the liver. Too much beta-carotene has been linked to a few problems:

▲ Liver damage

▲ Lung cancer in smokers

Excessive amounts of vitamin A (10,000 IU and above) can cause birth defects in pregnant women. This is because of its immediate availability to the body, whereas beta-carotene must first be converted to vitamin A in the body, lowering the risk of toxicity. Especially if you're pregnant, consider selecting a supplement containing beta-carotene rather than vitamin A.

VITAMIN B_1 (THIAMIN)

Thiamin, the common name for vitamin B_1, is the first of the lengthy list of B vitamins. Like the other Bs, it helps break down food for energy. It has other critical roles, as well.

THIAMIN'S ROLE IN YOUR BODY

Thiamin primarily helps break down carbohydrates, providing simpler sugars for your body to burn as energy. Vitamin B_1 also helps to maintain your nervous system. It may reduce symptoms of depression and accompanying memory loss, especially in older people.

RECOMMENDED DIETARY ALLOWANCES FOR VITAMIN B$_1$ (MG OF THIAMIN)

AGE	RDA
Infants 0–6 mos	0.3
Infants 6 mos–1 year	0.4
Children 1–3 years	0.7
Children 4–6 years	0.9
Children 7–10 years	1.0
Men 11–14 years	1.3
Men 15–18 years	1.5
Men 19–24 years	1.5
Men 25–50 years	1.5
Men 51+ years	1.4
Women 11–14 years	1.1
Women 15–18 years	1.1
Women 19–24 years	1.1
Women 25–50 years	1.1
Women 51+ years	1.0
Pregnant Women	1.5
Breastfeeding Women	1.6

A NOTE ABOUT THE Bs

Vitamin B is subdivided into many categories. In general, the B vitamins help your body break down carbohydrates, proteins, and fat. As a group, they may contribute to blood vessel health, relieve symptoms of stress and depression, and help keep your vision sharp. Each also has individual benefits, as well.

You'll find the B vitamins in any food product containing yeast and in many whole grains. Several of the Bs are added to foods, especially breads, cereals, and flour. Most of the B vitamins are found in multivitamin/multimineral supplements. A few of the B vitamins can be found in single supplements.

VITAMIN B$_2$ (RIBOFLAVIN)

Have you ever taken a multivitamin and then been shocked to see bright yellow urine? You can blame the neon color on riboflavin. But beyond turning your urine yellow, riboflavin is essential to your health.

RIBOFLAVIN'S ROLE IN YOUR BODY

Riboflavin, vitamin B$_2$'s most common name, helps break down fat. It has other roles within your body, as well:

▲ Helps cells use oxygen
▲ Lessens symptoms of depression
▲ Helps prevent cataracts
▲ Helps prevent eye fatigue

RECOMMENDED DIETARY ALLOWANCES
FOR VITAMIN B$_2$ (MG OF RIBOFLAVIN)

AGE	RDA
Infants 0–6 mos	0.4
Infants 6 mos–1 year	0.5
Children 1–3 years	0.8
Children 4–6 years	1.1
Children 7–10 years	1.2
Men 11–14 years	1.5
Men 15–18 years	1.8
Men 19–24 years	1.7
Men 25–50 years	1.7
Men 51+ years	1.4
Women 11–14 years	1.3
Women 15–18 years	1.3
Women 19–24 years	1.3
Women 25–50 years	1.3
Women 51+ years	1.2

RECOMMENDED DIETARY ALLOWANCES
FOR VITAMIN B₂ (MG OF RIBOFLAVIN) (CONTINUED)

AGE	RDA
Pregnant Women	1.6
Breastfeeding Women (first 6 months)	1.8
Breastfeeding Women (second 6 months)	1.7

VITAMIN B₃ (NIACIN OR NICOTINIC ACID)

Niacin is a B vitamin that has been used for many years at high doses as a medication for controlling high cholesterol. But its usefulness is not limited to its high-dose medication form. Even in smaller doses, niacin keeps you healthy in many ways.

NIACIN'S ROLE IN YOUR BODY

One of niacin's primary roles is to keep your blood vessels open. This has many benefits to your health. First off, niacin can help reduce "bad" LDL cholesterol and triglyceride and help raise "good" HDL cholesterol levels in your blood. Niacin can be so effective in this, that it can even help reverse artery disease. By keeping your blood flowing well, niacin has been linked to relieving inflammation and pain associated with arthritis.

There's more. Niacin also helps maintain the health of your nervous system. And it is involved in the process of creating hormones, chemicals that help your body perform many functions.

RECOMMENDED DIETARY ALLOWANCES
FOR VITAMIN B₃ (MG OF NIACIN)

AGE	RDA
Infants 0–6 mos	5
Infants 6 mos–1 year	6
Children 1–3 years	9
Children 4–6 years	12
Children 7–10 years	13
Men 11–14 years	17

RECOMMENDED DIETARY ALLOWANCES
FOR VITAMIN B$_3$ (MG OF NIACIN) (CONTINUED)

AGE	RDA
Men 15–18 years	20
Men 19–24 years	19
Men 25–50 years	19
Men 51+ years	15
Women 11–14 years	15
Women 15–18 years	15
Women 19–24 years	15
Women 25–50 years	15
Women 51+ years	13
Pregnant Women	17
Breastfeeding Women	20

CAUTIONS

Even a little bit of niacin (50 mg daily) can cause some side effects:

▲ Cramps

▲ Flushing

▲ Headaches

▲ Nausea

High doses of niacin (higher than 2000 mg daily) can cause serious problems:

▲ Irregular heartbeat

▲ High blood glucose

▲ Liver damage

Because of niacin's potential side effects, if you're taking high doses to lower cholesterol and fat levels, you should be consulting with a doctor.

VITAMIN B₅ (PANTOTHENIC ACID)

This lesser-known B vitamin has some interesting possibilities, beyond its primary role of breaking down food for energy. Pantothenic acid is involved in almost every process your body undertakes. It may also be responsible for reducing the amount of gray hair in those of us old enough to worry about that. There is no RDA for vitamin B₅.

VITAMIN B₆ (PYRIDOXINE)

Another "sleeper" that doesn't get a lot of attention, vitamin B₆ has a range of benefits to your health. Unfortunately, most people get only about half the RDA for pyridoxine.

VITAMIN B₆'s ROLE IN YOUR BODY

The range of effects vitamin B₆ has on the body is truly astounding. Vitamin B₆ helps you do the following:

- ▲ Digest and use proteins and fats
- ▲ Regulate sodium and potassium, the minerals that are responsible for maintaining a proper fluid balance in the body
- ▲ Lower your risk for artery disease
- ▲ Relieve symptoms of depression
- ▲ Maintain a strong immune system, by aiding the development of white blood cells (the cells that fight off infection)
- ▲ Maintain healthy skin
- ▲ Relieve symptoms of carpal tunnel syndrome

A deficit of vitamin B₆ may lead to artery problems, as this vitamin along with vitamin B₁₂ and folic acid help regulate homocysteine, a chemical in the blood that is linked to artery disease.

If you're over age 65, your body may not absorb B₆ as well as it did. As a result, you may need to take more of it in order to have an adequate amount.

RECOMMENDED DIETARY ALLOWANCES FOR VITAMIN B$_6$ (MG OF PYRIDOXINE)

AGE	RDA
Infants 0–6 mos	0.3
Infants 6 mos–1 year	0.6
Children 1–3 years	1.0
Children 4–6 years	1.1
Children 7-10 years	1.4
Men 11-14 years	1.7
Men 15 years and older	2.0
Women 11–14 years	1.4
Women 15–18 years	1.5
Women 19 years and older	1.6
Pregnant Women	2.2
Breastfeeding Women	2.1

CAUTIONS

Even though vitamin B$_6$ is sometimes used to limit symptoms of carpal tunnel syndrome, too much of it can cause these very same symptoms.

VITAMIN B$_{12}$

Vitamin B$_{12}$ works with many of the other B vitamins to maintain your health.

VITAMIN B$_{12}$'s ROLE IN YOUR BODY

Vitamin B$_{12}$ performs a myriad of tasks throughout your body. Here are some of them:

▲ Keeps the nervous system strong, and is sometimes recommended for people dealing with chronic fatigue syndrome

▲ Changes artery-damaging homocysteine into methionine, an amino acid with beneficial properties

▲ Reduces symptoms of depression, dementia, memory loss, and confusion

▲ Helps you think more clearly, even if you have no mental difficulties

A deficit in B_{12} can lead to the following problems:

▲ Impaired memory, to the point of mimicking senility

▲ An increase in homocysteine levels in the blood. Homocysteine is a chemical found in the blood that seems to contribute to artery disease and heart attacks.

RECOMMENDED DIETARY ALLOWANCES
FOR VITAMIN B_{12} (MCG)

AGE	RDA
Infants 0–6 mos	0.3
Infants 6 mos–1 year	0.5
Children 1–3 years	0.7
Children 4–6 years	1.0
Children 7–10 years	1.4
Men and Women 11 years and older	2.0
Pregnant Women	2.2
Breastfeeding Women	2.6

SOURCES OF VITAMIN B_{12}

Vitamin B_{12} is found mostly in animal products, including the following:

▲ Dairy products

▲ Eggs

SUPPLEMENTS

Increased intake of B_{12}—and possibly supplementation—is desirable in these circumstances:

▲ If you are a vegetarian and eat no animal products
▲ If you're over age 65, your body may not absorb B_{12} as well as it did

CAUTIONS

Because B_{12} is stored in the liver, excess amounts can cause liver damage.

Even a little alcohol (one to two drinks a day) can interfere with absorption of B_{12}.

VITAMIN B_{15} (PANGAMIC ACID)

This B vitamin helps break down food for energy. It also helps your blood carry oxygen throughout the body. There is no RDA for vitamin B_{15}.

BIOTIN

Even though it doesn't have a number or an RDA, it's still a B vitamin. Biotin helps break down fat for energy. It also benefits your hair, reducing both gray and hair loss. You'll frequently find biotin as an ingredient in hair care products such as shampoo.

FOLIC ACID (FOLATE OR FOLICIN)

Another B vitamin without a number, folic acid keeps making the news. For many years, the function of folic acid in the body was not well understood. In fact, several years ago scientists believed that the role of folic acid was so slight, that the RDA for folic acid was cut in half. But more recently, researchers have been discovering that this B vitamin plays many crucial roles—and that most of us probably need far more folic acid than we get each day.

FOLIC ACID'S ROLE IN YOUR BODY

Folic acid is the synthetic form of folate. Folate helps cells divide, a normal process that occurs constantly throughout your body. It also helps your body use iron, an essential ingredient in the production of the red blood cells that carry oxygen throughout your body. It only makes sense that because folate is such a key player in these basic processes, deficiencies in this nutrient are associated with many problems:

- ▲ Neural tube (brain and spinal cord) defects in a developing fetus. These defects include anencephaly (partial or missing brain leading to stillbirth or death shortly after birth), encephalocele (in which part of the brain protrudes or herniates), and spina bifida (in which the spine doesn't completely close up, leading to problems ranging from physical disability to mental retardation). Neural tube defects occur in about one or two of every 1000 births in the United States.
- ▲ Anemia

Besides simply not getting enough folic acid through diet, other causes can lead to folic acid deficiencies:

- ▲ Overuse of alcohol
- ▲ Smoking cigarettes
- ▲ Using oral contraceptives

Just as a deficit of folic acid can cause many health problems, many potential benefits result from adequate intake of folic acid:

- ▲ Prevention of as many as half of all neural tube defects in developing fetuses.
- ▲ A decrease in risk for cardiovascular disease, including heart attacks and stroke. Folic acid seems to affect homocysteine, a chemical associated with artery disease when found in high levels in the blood. Folic acid changes homocysteine into a harmless amino acid. This reduced risk occurs even for those who have a genetic predisposition for artery disease.

▲ Possibly reduced risk for colorectal, cervical, and lung cancer
▲ Reduced symptoms of dementia and depression
▲ Improvement of concentration and memory, even in healthy people.

RECOMMENDED DIETARY ALLOWANCES
FOR FOLATE (MCG)

AGE	RDA
Infants 0–6 mos	25
Infants 6 mos–1 year	35
Children 1–3 years	50
Children 4–6 years	75
Children 7–10 years	100
Men 11–14 years	150
Men 15 years and older	200
Women 11–14 years	150
Women 15 years and older	180
Pregnant Women	400
Breastfeeding Women (first 6 months)	280
Breastfeeding Women (second 6 months)	260

These RDAs are likely to be raised soon—probably more than doubled for most of us. In the meanwhile, most nutrition experts recommend that women who have the possibility of becoming pregnant—that is, women between the ages of 15 and 45—should probably get 0.4 mg (400 mcg) of folic acid every day. This ensures that if you become pregnant—even accidentally—the fetus will have enough folic acid in the earliest days of development, when most defects are likely to occur. Children over the age of 4 and adult men should also have 400 mcg of folic acid each day. It is expected that the RDA for pregnant women will double to 800 mcg of folic acid daily.

It may be difficult to eat enough food to meet the RDA for folic acid, making supplementation a wise choice. Supplementation may be especially helpful in the winter, when fresh fruits and vegetables are less available.

The maximum safe level for folic acid is 1000 mcg (1 mg) per day.

SOURCES OF FOLIC ACID

Folic acid can be found in many foods:

- ▲ Chickpeas, black-eyed peas, kidney beans, lentils, lima beans, navy beans, pinto beans, and other dried beans
- ▲ Cheese
- ▲ Citrus fruits, such as grapefruit and oranges
- ▲ Leafy green vegetables such as asparagus, broccoli, Brussels sprouts, collard greens, romaine lettuce, spinach, and turnip greens
- ▲ Meat (especially liver), fish, and poultry
- ▲ Wheat germ
- ▲ Whole grains

Because of the critical role of this nutrient, you'll now find folic acid added to breads, cereal, pasta, flour, and other grain products.

SUPPLEMENTS

In some studies, supplements lowered risk of cardiovascular disease slightly more than simply eating foods high in folic acid. Supplementation may be especially important for older people, who tend to have lower intake of foods high in folic acid and who may also have more difficulty in absorbing this nutrient. Supplementation is also recommended for women who may become or who are already pregnant.

Supplements may claim on the label to help reduce neural tube birth defects if the product provides at least ten percent of the RDA for folic acid, and does not contain more than one hundred percent of the RDA for vitamins A and D (for which high doses are linked to birth defects). If it contains more than one hundred percent of the RDA for folic acid, it must note that 1000 mcg of folic acid is the maximum safe level.

CAUTIONS

Taking high amounts of folic acid—over 1000 mcg (1 mg) daily—may hide deficiencies of vitamin B_{12}, especially in older adults. It may also make some anticancer drugs and epilepsy drugs less effective.

Drinking even moderate amounts of alcohol (one to two drinks a day) may interfere somewhat with the absorption of folic acid.

LECITHIN (PHOSPHATIDYLCHOLINE OR PC)

Lecithin is sometimes considered to be a B vitamin. It helps break down fat and protects your nerves, among other things. It may help relieve symptoms associated with Alzheimer's disease. It may also help lower cholesterol. There is no RDA for lecithin.

PARA-AMINO BENZOIC ACID (PABA)

The last of the B vitamins, PABA is perhaps best known as the active ingredient in sunscreen. It does more than protect you from UV rays. PABA also helps your body form folic acid. It may help prevent gray hair. There is no RDA for PABA.

VITAMIN C

Vitamin C holds the distinction of being the first of the vitamins to be discovered. But even though it has been known about the longest, it continues to bring surprises to researchers, who are still finding new uses for vitamin C in the body. Most scientists don't believe the scientist Linus Pauling's claims that taking high doses of vitamin C could not only cure a cold, but add twelve to eighteen years to your life. Who's to argue with a man who lived actively into his nineties? But even if you don't agree totally with Dr. Pauling, vitamin C is still an amazing nutrient. The sad truth is, though, that despite its well-established value to health, about half of us don't meet even the minimum RDA for vitamin C—even though simply eating an orange a day would do the trick.

VITAMIN C'S ROLE IN YOUR BODY

Practically everyone knows the importance of getting enough vitamin C, after it made headlines for limiting symptoms of the common cold. Vitamin C works against colds in a couple of ways:

- ▲ It strengthens your body's immune response to the types of viruses that cause colds.
- ▲ If you catch a cold, it works as a mild antihistamine, helping to block the action of the hormone histamine, which causes the nasal stuffiness often associated with colds.

But besides treating colds, why else is vitamin C so critical? Most important, vitamin C simply helps your cells burn energy. But besides this vital, ongoing function, there's a long list of the benefits of vitamin C. Let's start with the immune system, for which vitamin C serves effectively as:

- ▲ A general immune system booster, protecting you from many other "foreign" and internal threats
- ▲ Protection from viruses such as pneumonia

But the benefits continue. Vitamin C plays a vital role in maintaining the health of your blood vessels, including those in your heart.

- ▲ Helps prevent heart and artery disease
- ▲ Lowers "bad" LDL cholesterol levels in your blood vessels and may even raise "good" HDL cholesterol levels in some people
- ▲ May help lower your blood pressure, especially if you're a smoker

The net result is a decreased risk for high blood pressure, artery problems, heart attacks, and stroke.

Vitamin C also provides benefits in relation to cancer, a category of diseases in which damaged cells in an organ multiply out of control:

- ▲ Helps prevent many forms of cancer
- ▲ Has been used to help relieve symptoms from cancer chemotherapies, and may be an effective chemotherapy itself
- ▲ May protect against cancer-causing food additives (nitrates and nitrites)

Vitamin C also plays a big role in maintaining the health of your eyes:

- ▲ Helps prevent cataracts, a clouding of the lens of the eye
- ▲ May help control glaucoma, a disease in which the pressure inside the eye is too high and fluid cannot drain from the eye properly
- ▲ May help prevent macular degeneration, an eye disease in which the part of your eye that focuses light for your central vision is damaged

In addition, vitamin C has other benefits:

- ▲ May improve sperm's quality and motility (ability to move around), especially in men who smoke
- ▲ Helps block UV light, preventing premature aging of the skin, while still allowing the light to interact with the skin to produce vitamin D
- ▲ May help reduce signs of aging in the skin

A deficit of vitamin C can lead to scurvy, a disease that routinely led to the deaths of sailors who had no fresh fruits or vegetables during long voyages. Symptoms of scurvy include bleeding of the gums and under the skin, loss of teeth, general weakness and depression, and slow healing of wounds.

RECOMMENDED DIETARY ALLOWANCES FOR VITAMIN C (MG)

AGE	WEIGHT	RDA
Infants 0–6 mos	(13 lbs)	30
Infants 6 mos–1 year	(20 lbs)	35
Children 1–3 years	(29 lbs)	40
Children 4–6 years	(44 lbs)	45
Children 7–10 years	(52 lbs)	45
Men and Women 11–14 years		50
Men and Women 15 years and older		60
Pregnant Women		70
Breastfeeding Women (first 6 months)		95
Breastfeeding Women (second 6 months)		90

There has been some discussion about raising the RDA for vitamin C to about 200 mg. Daily doses up to about 250 mg seem to provide the greatest health benefits. However, increasing the dose above that level doesn't bring as many benefits. And after 500 mg or so, most of the vitamin C you take is simply excreted out through urine.

If you smoke, your body may be depleted of vitamin C. In addition, the damage caused by smoking may increase your need for vitamin C even more—the RDA for smokers is 100 mg (60 mg for nonsmokers). You may want to consider supplementation.

SOURCES OF VITAMIN C

Your body cannot make vitamin C itself, so your entire supply must come from external sources, either through food or supplements. Most fruits and vegetables contain at least some vitamin C. The following are especially good sources of vitamin C:

- ▲ Broccoli
- ▲ Cauliflower
- ▲ Citrus (oranges, grapefruit, lemons)

- ▲ Papaya
- ▲ Potatoes
- ▲ Spinach and other green, leafy vegetables
- ▲ Strawberries

SUPPLEMENTS

Not enough research has been done to determine if long-term supplementation of vitamin C above the RDA level poses any threat to your health.

Chewing many vitamin C tablets can be hard on your teeth—the acids that make up vitamin C are corrosive. Consider taking tablets that you swallow.

CAUTIONS

Contrary to popular belief, too much vitamin C can cause problems, even though most of the excess is excreted out through the urine. Overdoses of vitamin C are associated with several symptoms:

- ▲ Cramps and diarrhea
- ▲ Kidney stones
- ▲ Interfering with urine glucose test results

VITAMIN D

Spend just 15 minutes in the sun, and you probably have met your RDA for vitamin D. How can that happen? And why might you need a supplement, too?

VITAMIN D'S ROLE IN YOUR BODY

When you think of nutrients related to bones, the first nutrient that probably comes to mind is calcium. But without vitamin D, your body cannot use calcium to maintain strong bones. Vitamin D helps you use calcium in a couple of ways. First, it helps your body absorb calcium from the digestive tract. Then vitamin D helps calcium to become deposited in two storage areas: your bones and teeth.

A deficit of vitamin D can lead to bone problems such as rickets (bowlegs or knock-knees from improper bone development) in children. It can also contribute to the development of osteoporosis (weakening of bones), broken bones, and osteomalacia (soft bones) in adults.

Besides helping to maintain strong bones and teeth, vitamin D has also been linked to lowering your risk for certain cancers, including breast cancer.

RECOMMENDED DIETARY
ALLOWANCES FOR VITAMIN D (MCG)

AGE	WEIGHT	RDA
Infants 0–6 mos	(13 lbs)	7.5
Infants 6 mos–1 year	(20 lbs)	10
Children 1–10 years		10
Men 11–24 years		10
Men 25 years and older		5
Women 11–24 years		10
Women 25 years and older		5
Pregnant and Breastfeeding Women		10

Even though the "official" RDAs for vitamin D are lower, most experts recommend 200 IU (20 mcg). For older adults, most doctors recommend 400–800 IU of vitamin D.

SOURCES OF VITAMIN D

Believe it or not, the sun is the primary source of vitamin D. The sun's ultraviolet (**UV**) rays are absorbed into your skin, initiating a complex reaction involving the skin, liver, and kidneys that eventually transforms chemicals in your skin into vitamin D. Ten to fifteen minutes of sun each day should help you meet the RDA for vitamin D. The darker your skin, the more sunlight you need. And sunscreens that block UV rays also prevent you from getting vitamin D.

An inactive form of vitamin D is naturally found in some foods:

▲ Butter

▲ Egg yolks

▲ Fatty fish (salmon, herring, and mackerel are examples)

Like with sunlight, the liver and kidneys convert this inactive form of the vitamin into a form your body can use.

Vitamin D is also routinely added to milk (two cups meet the current RDA for vitamin D), margarine, and many cereals.

SUPPLEMENTS

Vitamin D is one of the few nutrients for which most scientists and medical professionals recommend supplements. You may want to consider a vitamin D supplement if you:

▲ Are over age 55 (your body may not absorb vitamin D through sunlight and food as well as it did when you were younger and your bones may be beginning to break down more rapidly at this age).

▲ Have limited exposure to sunlight.

▲ Don't drink milk.

▲ Have a disease that prevents your body from absorbing or processing vitamin D in adequate quantities (kidney and liver problems and digestive disorders that prevent absorption of fat can all inhibit use of vitamin D).

▲ Take certain medications such as phentoin (**Dilatin**) used to treat heart problems and epilepsy.

CAUTIONS

You should probably not take more than 400 IU of vitamin D each day unless prescribed by or monitored by a doctor. Because excess amounts are stored in body fat, vitamin D can become toxic. Taking too much of this vitamin—more than 2000 IU daily—can lead to several serious problems:

▲ Irritability

▲ Nausea, headache, and weight loss

▲ Excessive urination and kidney damage

▲ High blood pressure

▲ Calcium deposits in your kidneys and lungs

If you are taking a calcium supplement as well, make sure that it doesn't already contain vitamin D. Many do, since calcium needs vitamin D to be used by the body. Don't accidentally double-dose.

VITAMIN E (ALPHA-TOCOPHEROL)

Preached as the latest wonder drug, vitamin E has been hyped to do everything from curing cancer to preventing aging. Although these claims may seem farfetched, there is some underlying truth to them. Vitamin E is an amazing substance.

VITAMIN E'S ROLE IN YOUR BODY

Vitamin E is probably the most studied of the antioxidants. It does seem to help disable the free radicals responsible for damage to the skin, the heart, the arteries, and some organs such as the eyes. Vitamin E has less dramatic but equally important roles as well, including the following:

▲ Helping to form red blood cells, the cells that carry oxygen through your blood

▲ Helping your nervous system work properly

▲ Improving the immune system's response to foreign substances, especially in people over age 65

Concerning cardiovascular health, a review of many studies shows that people who have a high level of vitamin E in their blood have fewer problems with artery and heart disease. It seems that vitamin E latches onto the "bad" LDL cholesterol in your blood, keeping it from piling up against the artery walls.

Vitamin E helps people with digestive disorders that affect the absorption of nutrients from their digestive systems. It has also been used with premature infants. Vitamin E may also play a role in other areas:

- ▲ Preventing baldness
- ▲ Preventing cataracts
- ▲ Slowing the effects of Parkinson's and Alzheimer's diseases
- ▲ Reducing symptoms of fibrocystic breast disease

RECOMMENDED DIETARY ALLOWANCES
FOR VITAMIN E (MG OF ALPHA-TOCOPHEROL)

AGE	WEIGHT	RDA
Infants 0–6 mos	(13 lbs)	3
Infants 6 mos–1 year	(20 lbs)	4
Children 1–3 years	(29 lbs)	6
Children 4–6 years	(44 lbs)	7
Children 7–10 years	(52 lbs)	7
Men 11 years and older		10
Women 11 years and older		8
Pregnant Women		10
Breastfeeding Women (first 6 months)		12
Breastfeeding Women (second 6 months)		11

Many nutrition experts recommend 12 IU (12 mg) for women, 15 IU (15 mg) for men.

SOURCES OF VITAMIN E

You'll find vitamin E in the following types of foods:

- ▲ Green, leafy vegetables
- ▲ Nuts
- ▲ Oils
- ▲ Wheat germ

SUPPLEMENTS

No one has determined adequate levels for additional supplementation of vitamin E. Many studies have used 400–1000 IU (400-1000 mg) for supplementation. Some experts recommend that if you're over age 65, you could benefit from an additional 200 IU (200 mg) of vitamin E daily.

CAUTIONS

Not enough research has been done to determine if long-term supplementation of vitamin E above the RDA level has any health risks associated with it. It is known that supplementation above 1080 IU can lead to stomach problems.

You should be careful about using vitamin E if you take any blood-thinning medications such as warfarin (**Coumadin**). Bleeding may occur.

VITAMIN K

One of the "forgotten" vitamins, nevertheless vitamin K plays an important role in the body.

VITAMIN K'S ROLE IN YOUR BODY

Many people are aware that vitamin K helps blood to clot. In fact, if you take blood-thinning medication, you probably have a supply of vitamin K on hand in case your blood becomes too thin and you begin bleeding or hemorrhaging. In addition, vitamin K is often used as an antidote to certain poisonous substances that cause uncontrolled internal bleeding.

But did you know that vitamin K plays a critical role in bone health, too? It activates certain proteins that are involved in the process of forming new bone. In fact, researchers are now convinced that vitamin K's worth has been underestimated and that the RDA needs to be raised.

A deficiency in vitamin K is associated with these problems:

▲ Blood that doesn't clot properly

▲ Lower bone density in adults of all ages, both men and women

RECOMMENDED DIETARY ALLOWANCES FOR VITAMIN K (MCG)

AGE	WEIGHT	RDA
Infants 0–6 mos	(13 lbs)	5
Infants 6 mos–1 year	(20 lbs)	10
Children 1–3 years	(29 lbs)	15
Children 4–6 years	(44 lbs)	20
Children 7–10 years	(52 lbs)	30
Men 11–14 years	(99 lbs)	45
Men 15–18 years	(145 lbs)	65
Men 19–24 years	(160 lbs)	70
Men 25–50 years	(174 lbs)	80
Men 51+ years	(170 lbs)	80
Women 11–14 years	(101 lbs)	45
Women 15–18 years	(120 lbs)	55
Women 19–24 years	(128 lbs)	60
Women 25–50 years	(138 lbs)	65
Women 51+ years	(143 lbs)	65
Pregnant and Breastfeeding Women		65

Most experts recommend 85 to 95 mcg daily, the amount needed for normal blood clotting. Most of us easily get this level of vitamin K through our diets, except for people from ages 25 to 30.

SOURCES OF VITAMIN K

Vitamin K is associated with the plant chemical, chlorophyll. So the best source of the vitamin is anything that has a lot of chlorophyll in it—the greener, the better. You'll find plenty of vitamin K in these items:

- ▲ Broccoli, collard greens, spinach, and other leafy, green vegetables
- ▲ Vegetable oils such as canola, olive, and soybean (not corn or peanut oil)
- ▲ Products containing a lot of these vegetable oils, such as salad dressings

SUPPLEMENTS

Most people easily meet the current RDA for vitamin K through their diets. However, there is some talk of raising the RDA for vitamin K even higher to prevent more bone problems. You may want to consider this, especially if you're at risk for developing bone problems.

VITAMIN Q

See Coenzyme Q-10 in Chapter 4.

CHAPTER 3

Minerals

Minerals are everywhere. You'll find them all around you. They are in soil, plants, and rocks. They are in your body. So how do they get in our food? How do they get in our bodies? Why do we even need minerals?

Minerals are naturally occurring substances with a definite chemical composition and specific characteristics in shape, color, and hardness. Minerals are essential to the life of all plants and animals—including humans. You may be surprised at the huge amount of work that minerals perform in your body. Minerals play a large part in your ability to think and eat, allowing your body to function smoothly, quickly, and accurately by completing your body's nutritional requirements.

But don't go outside, scoop up a spoonful of dirt, and put it on your breakfast cereal. Just like anything you put into your body, you need to be vigilant about minerals—the amounts of and quality of them. So how does the mineral "food chain" occur? Minerals occur naturally on the earth in rocks and soil. Plants grow in the soil. Animals come along and eat the plants. Humans eat both the plants and the animals that have eaten the plants. This is the natural way for minerals to make their way into your body.

THE ROLE OF MINERALS IN YOUR BODY

Your body utilizes at least twenty different minerals to perform its various functions. Here are just a few examples of how your body benefits from minerals:

- ▲ A healthy, strong immune system
- ▲ Cancer prevention

▲ Coherent thinking processes

▲ Formation and maintenance of bones and teeth

▲ A strong, regular heartbeat

All of these functions are influenced, for good or for ill, by minerals.

MACRO-AND MICROMINERALS IN YOUR BODY

There are at least twenty different minerals found in the human body: calcium, chloride, chromium, cobalt, copper, fluoride, iodine, iron, magnesium, manganese, molybdenum, nickel, phosphorus, potassium, selenium, silicon, sodium, sulfur, vanadium, and zinc. Little is know about these minerals. The others can be broken down into two categories. Macrominerals are needed in the largest amounts, although that does not necessarily mean they are the most important. Macrominerals include:

▲ Calcium

▲ Magnesium

▲ Sodium

▲ Potassium

▲ Phosphorus

Microminerals, otherwise called trace minerals, include the following:

▲ Boron

▲ Chromium

▲ Copper

▲ Iodine

▲ Iron

▲ Manganese

▲ Selenium

▲ Zinc

In addition, although flouride is not technically a mineral, we have included information about this vital nutrient in this section.

This chapter will discuss specific information for each of these minerals, including what each mineral does in your body and symptoms associated with both deficiencies and overuse. We will give any RDAs that have been established, as well as provide information about other recommendations and cautions for mineral use.

MINERAL DEFICIENCIES

With our wide-ranging food supply, it is amazing that so many of us are lacking in the basic elements our bodies need for good health. There are many reasons for mineral deficiencies:

- ▲ We overcook our foods.
- ▲ We use too much water to cook our foods.
- ▲ We strenuously exercise.
- ▲ We eat processed foods.
- ▲ We diet.
- ▲ We eat high-fat foods.
- ▲ We smoke.
- ▲ We drink alcohol.
- ▲ We take prescription and over-the-counter medications.

The end result of any of these practices can be a mineral deficiency. Overcooking foods destroys minerals. Cooking in too much water causes minerals to leach out of the food. Highly processed foods lose minerals during the processing stages. A low-calorie diet may not allow you to fit in everything you need for adequate mineral intake. High-fat foods are generally low in mineral content and may make you feel full, leaving you without the desire to eat more nutritional foods. Smoking uses up your store of minerals more quickly. Drinking excessive alcohol impairs your liver function, increasing the possibility of losing vital minerals. Prescription and over-the-counter medications may counteract the effectiveness of minerals in your body, or in the case of diuretics (water pills), minerals may be eliminated from your body before being utilized.

Who is most at risk for having mineral deficiencies? One recent study shows that teenage girls, from age 14 to 16, were below the RDA standards for the greatest number of minerals. Women between the ages 25 and 30, adults between ages 60 to 65, and children below the age of 2 also tend to be under the RDA recommendations for several minerals.

MINERAL TOXICITY

The RDAs were established to give us the minimum amount of minerals we need on a daily basis. But what is the amount needed to optimize your health and prevent disease? That optimal amount varies for each mineral, and is not even always known. Because excess minerals are stored in your body for future use in your bones and muscle tissues, it is possible to build up a toxic amount. This is especially true for older people with iron. Do not take more than the recommended amounts of minerals for your age and gender group unless you are being monitored by a health care practitioner who is knowledgeable about mineral supplementation.

WHEN TO SUPPLEMENT

Mineral supplements should never be used instead of a healthy diet. But even many dietitians today have come to the conclusion that if you stick to the recommended number of calories in your diet, it may be difficult to include all the minerals you need for good health. For instance, would you like to eat at least five bananas a day? That's the amount needed to get the optimal amount of potassium into your system to prevent or manage high blood pressure. If you need to restrict your calories to control or maintain appropriate weight, mineral supplementation may be appropriate. It may also be helpful if you are older (you may need increased supplies or your body may absorb minerals less readily). There are other reasons to supplement with specific minerals, which are discussed as needed in the descriptions that follow.

BORON

Boron, a micromineral, was discovered in the 1900s, but evidence of it in the human body wasn't discovered until the mid-1980s.

BORON'S ROLE IN YOUR BODY

One of the primary functions of boron is to assist in the breakdown of calcium, magnesium, and phosphorus. Boron works with calcium, magnesium, and vitamin D in helping new bone growth, possibly preventing osteoporosis. Osteoporosis results in brittle, weak bones that break easily. There is evidence that boron helps build muscle and enhances brain functions.

A study of post-menopausal women taking 3 mg of boron daily resulted in a forty percent reduction in calcium loss through urination, thirty-three percent less magnesium loss, and the participants also lost lesser amounts of phosphorus.

A boron deficiency may result in decreased levels of calcium, phosphorus, and magnesium.

RECOMMENDED DIETARY ALLOWANCES FOR BORON

There is no RDA for boron at this time. Most experts recommend that supplements stay within the 1.5 mg to 3 mg range.

SOURCES OF BORON

Boron can be found in apples, carrots, nuts, and grapes.

SUPPLEMENTS

The elderly may benefit the most from using a boron supplement. They often have difficulty absorbing enough calcium—boron may reduce calcium loss through urination.

CAUTIONS

Excessive boron may result in diarrhea, nausea, and skin rashes.

CALCIUM

Calcium is the most abundant macromineral found in your body. Ninety-nine percent of the calcium in your body is found in your bones and teeth, while the remaining calcium is found in your blood and other body fluids. Calcium intake daily should be around 1,200–1,500 mg, but studies show most people only include approximately 500–600 mg, or roughly half the amount your body should be receiving.

CALCIUM'S ROLE IN YOUR BODY

Why is calcium so important? Calcium is instrumental in reducing the rate of bone loss—protecting you from osteoporosis, a disease that makes your bones brittle and weak, often resulting in fractures and a stooped-over posture. Calcium also helps the nervous system to function properly by helping the release of the neurotransmitters that carry messages from one nerve cell to another. It is needed for blood clotting, which helps wounds heal faster. Calcium is required for maintaining a healthy blood pressure by helping to break down fats and by possibly helping the body to excrete excess sodium. Low consumption of calcium has been shown to increase your risk of developing high blood pressure. It is also believed that calcium helps to prevent colon cancer from developing. Combine a low amount of vitamin D with a low amount of calcium and your risk for breast cancer increases.

SOURCES OF CALCIUM

Dairy products provide approximately fifty-five percent of your daily calcium intake. If you are not eating or drinking enough dairy products, it is extremely difficult to work in enough calcium into your diet through food. For example, you would need to eat 5–6 cups of cooked broccoli just to equal three servings of dairy products.

Calcium is found in the following foods:

- ▲ Dairy products
- ▲ Seaweed

- Sardines
- Green leafy vegetables
- Meat, poultry, and eggs
- Calcium-fortified orange juice
- Broccoli
- Cooked dried beans and peas

Alcohol, coffee, sugars, and some medications can keep your body from absorbing all of the calcium you eat.

RECOMMENDED DIETARY ALLOWANCES FOR CALCIUM (MG)

AGE	RDA
Infants 0–6 mos	400
Infants 6 mos–1 year	600
Children 1–3 years	800
Children 4–6 years	800
Children 7–10 years	800
Men and Women 11–14 years	1200
Men and Women 15–18 years	1200
Men and Women 19–24 years	1200
Men and Women 25–50 years	800
Men and Women 51+ years	800
Pregnant and Breastfeeding Women	1200

SUPPLEMENTS

Calcium can be a tricky mineral supplement to take properly—if you take too much at one time, your body can't absorb all of the calcium in a timely fashion and excretes the leftover amount. In addition, calcium is absorbed better when you have adequate amounts of other nutrients, including boron, lysine, magnesium, manganese, phosphorus, and vitamins A, C, and D. See descriptions of these nutrients elsewhere in this book. Calcium supplements have also been known to cause stomach upset, namely gas, so follow the directions on the label for the best time to take it.

Many antacid products contain low doses of calcium. However, these antacids may not provide you with enough calcium, and you may choose to take a calcium supplement. In some stores, there are more than twenty different types and brands of calcium. Remember, if you include a lot of calcium-rich foods in your diet, you may be able to take an antacid with calcium instead of purchasing the more expensive calcium supplements.

Calcium supplements are available in many forms. The two most popular and widely used are calcium carbonate and calcium citrate. The lesser used forms are calcium phosphate, calcium lactate, and calcium gluconate.

Calcium carbonate is one of the most commonly found and used forms of calcium supplement currently on the market. It comes in a highly concentrated form, allowing you to take fewer tablets each day. However, it has been known to cause both excessive gas and constipation in some people. Calcium carbonate neutralizes stomach acid, which can impair digestion by not allowing food to be broken down properly. Bacteria often takes over the breaking-down process, creating methane gas—accounting for the bloating, cramping feeling.

If you choose to give calcium carbonate a try, don't ever take it on an empty stomach. Take with or after a meal. Calcium carbonate also may not be absorbed as well as other forms of calcium. Splitting the dosage into two or more doses taken throughout the day will increase absorption while lowering stomach irritation.

Calcium citrate is another popular form of calcium. It is also available in powdered form, for those who have difficulty swallowing a pill or capsule. Calcium citrate is believed to be the best-absorbed form of calcium. It also does not have to be taken with meals and most people do not experience any stomach upset taking this form of calcium. However, calcium citrate is not as concentrated, so you will need to take more of it each day.

Calcium phosphate is also available in a highly concentrated form. Since it is difficult for your body to break down this form of calcium, you may be wisest to choose another form.

Calcium lactate and calcium gluconate are not available in highly concentrated forms. To get the same amount of calcium as the other forms, you need to take as many as six pills every day. For many people this is not very convenient, so you may wish to try a different form of calcium.

CAUTIONS

Whatever form of calcium you choose, make sure you are not taking more than 500 mg at one time. Taking more is like burning your money. Your body only can absorb about 500 mg of calcium at one time and will simply excrete the leftover calcium instead of holding it for future use.

CHROMIUM

Chromium is a trace micromineral that has been making a lot of news lately. There are claims that it will help you lose weight and build muscle. Although there is probably some truth to these claims, it is not a miracle mineral and should be used wisely. Realistically, these claims are probably only true in people who have a deficient amount of chromium in their bodies. For those who have a sufficient amount of chromium, the extra chromium isn't likely to cause you to lose a lot of weight or build up your muscles, but may decrease the effectiveness of insulin.

Approximately ninety percent of American diets are low in chromium intake. Your body has the highest amount of chromium during your infant years, then declines with age as you take in less chromium in your diet.

CHROMIUM'S ROLE IN YOUR BODY

Chromium's main function is to help insulin transfer glucose (a simple sugar) from your blood into your cells. By lowering blood sugar levels, chromium may help prevent diabetes, especially in people who are glucose intolerant. Chromium may also prevent diabetics from developing heart disease.

Although a chromium deficiency so low that it causes obvious problems is rare, many people have lower amounts of chromium than they should and may find supplements beneficial. If you experience numbness or tingling in your toes and fingers, reduced muscle coordination, or an increase in blood sugar levels, you may be chromium-deficient.

Low chromium levels in older adults are thought to be a contributing factor in a high incidence of diabetes in this age group. Low chromium levels are also associated with high cholesterol, which increases your risk for heart disease.

RECOMMENDED DIETARY ALLOWANCES FOR CHROMIUM

Currently there are no RDAs for chromium.

SOURCES OF CHROMIUM

Chromium is found naturally in some foods. You can include chromium in your diet by eating the following foods:

- ▲ Whole grains
- ▲ Fruits
- ▲ Vegetables

SUPPLEMENTS

There is currently no RDA recommendation for how much chromium you should be getting. There seems to be a consensus, though, that a range of 50–200 mcg should be a safe amount to take. If you are diabetic, overweight, or are physically inactive, ask your health care provider if you might benefit from taking chromium at the high end of the dosage scale.

CAUTIONS

Excessive chromium is thought to inhibit insulin's effectiveness. Let your health care provider know if you are taking chromium and are diabetic.

There is also a chance that high chromium levels may encourage the growth of an existing cancerous tumor.

COPPER

Copper is a micromineral found in all of your tissues, but primarily in the brain, heart, kidneys, and liver. Although a trace mineral, copper plays an important part in many body functions.

COPPER'S ROLE IN YOUR BODY

Copper is important in the development and maintenance of red blood cells, while guarding against anemia and bone deterioration. Copper is involved in many facets of the cardiovascular system—the heart, arteries, blood vessels—and the nervous system. Copper releases iron from storage, increasing the intestinal absorption of iron. It also breaks down fat tissue, which is needed to aid the normal functions of insulin. Copper plays a part in the conversion of your food—protein, carbohydrates, and fat—into energy for your use. Copper is beneficial to guard against cancer. It is thought to play a part in maintaining myelin, the protective sheaths surrounding your nerves, which may protect you from getting multiple sclerosis.

COPPER DEFICIENCY

Large dosages of vitamin C or the prolonged use of antacids may contribute to a copper deficiency. A severe copper deficiency is rare, most commonly found in malnourished children. Copper deficiency can cause anemia, arthritis, heart disease, high cholesterol, heart irregularities, and high blood sugar. These conditions raise your risk for heart attack.

But even a marginal copper deficiency, which is more common, can cause many of the same symptoms. Anemia, loss of color from the hair and skin, poor concentration, and numbness and tingling can result form a slight copper deficiency. A deficiency can also reduce the number of white blood cells, which increases your risk of catching an infectious disease.

RECOMMENDED DIETARY ALLOWANCES FOR COPPER

There are no current RDAs for copper.

SOURCES OF COPPER

Copper can be found in the following foods:

▲ Mushrooms

▲ Whole-grain and multi-grain breads and wheat germ

- Legumes
- Dried fruits
- Bananas
- Lean meats and liver
- Honey and molasses
- Hazelnuts, Brazil nuts, and walnuts
- Kelp

Unfortunately, many of these foods aren't normally on an everyday food plan. Plus only approximately thirty percent of all copper that you eat is actually absorbed by your body! It's easy to see why so many people are low on their copper intake.

SUPPLEMENTS

Copper can be found in many multivitamin/multimineral supplements. Several other nutrients aid in copper absorption, including folic acid, iron, and zinc. See the descriptions for these nutrients elsewhere in this book.

FLUORIDE

Fluoride is an element found along with minerals. It is technically neither a macro- or micromineral. Fluoride resides primarily in bones and teeth within the body.

FLUORIDE'S ROLE IN YOUR BODY

Fluoride's primary role is to protect the natural development of teeth. Fluoride also protects mature teeth from decay and the resulting cavities. Fluoride helps make bones strong, thereby helping to prevent osteoporosis—a disease that results in brittle, weak bones and fractures.

Elderly people may benefit from fluoride—it has been shown to reduce calcium excretion in urine, thus protecting bones from osteoporosis.

RECOMMENDED DIETARY ALLOWANCES FOR FLUORIDE

There is no RDA for fluoride. Most communities try to provide 1.5 mg to 4 mg per resident per day through fluoridated water.

SOURCES OF FLUORIDE

The primary source for fluoride supplementation is in fluoridated water. Many communities add fluoride to the water supplies. In addition, fluoride may be found in many pre-packaged beverages and foods due to fluoride from water used during production of the product. Some fluoride may be swallowed when brushing teeth with a fluoride toothpaste.

SUPPLEMENTS

If the community you live in has fluoridated water, you probably do not need extra fluoride supplements. If the water in your area does not contain fluoride, extra fluoride can be found in toothpaste and mouth rinses. A health care provider or dental health care provider may be able to provide you with a prescription for fluoride.

CAUTIONS

Some water naturally contains high levels of fluoride. Excessive fluoride may result in pitted teeth. It may even be fatal in some cases.

IODINE

Iodine is another micromineral found in your body. Back in the 1920s, some cities experimented with adding iodine to their water supplies. Even back then, it was realized that an iodine deficiency could cause goiter, which is an enlargement of the thyroid gland.

ROLE OF IODINE IN YOUR BODY

Iodine protects against goiter and is used by the thyroid gland to produce the hormone thyroxine. Thyroxine regulates energy production in the body. Iodine is involved in metabolizing excess fat, breaking it down to use as energy.

An iodine deficiency in adults may lead to breast cancer. In children, an iodine deficiency may lead to mental retardation. If you experience a metallic taste in your mouth, mouth sores, swollen salivary glands, diarrhea, and vomiting, you may want to have your iodine level checked.

RECOMMENDED DIETARY ALLOWANCES
FOR IODINE (MCG)

AGE	RDA
Infants 0–6 mos	40
Infants 6 mos–1 year	50
Children 1–3 years	70
Children 4–6 years	90
Children 7–10 years	120
Men and Women 11 years and older	150
Pregnant Women	175
Breastfeeding Women	200

SOURCES OF IODINE

Fortunately, iodized salt ensures most of us of getting enough iodine into our systems. These foods can also help ensure an adequate iodine level:

▲ Salt-water fish, lobster, and cooked oysters

▲ Garlic

▲ Lima beans and soybeans

▲ Mushrooms

▲ Sesame seeds

SUPPLEMENTS

For years, iodine supplements probably were not necessary. If you're on a salt-restricted diet, however, iodine supplementation should be considered.

CAUTIONS

One potential problem is that some foods, when consumed uncooked in large amounts, effectively block the absorption of iodine into your body. Brussels sprouts, cabbage, cauliflower, kale, peaches, pears, spinach, and turnips all may block iodine absorption and so should probably be eaten in moderate amounts only.

IRON

Iron is one of the body's microminerals, although an important mineral to your good health. Many ancient civilizations knew the benefits of iron. After battles, the Greeks, amongst others, fed their soldiers liver to speed their recovery from injuries. Then in the 1940s, the United States began fortifying food with vitamins and minerals—including iron.

IRON'S ROLE IN YOUR BODY

There are many reasons to make sure you are getting enough iron in your body. Iron helps protect you against heart disease, cancer, and neurological disorders—including multiple sclerosis. Iron plays an important role in energy production. Iron is a necessary component of hemoglobin, which carries oxygen to the cells and increases cells' immunity.

Iron deficiency causes muscle weakness, anemia, and decreased mental skills—including mood swings and memory loss. An iron deficiency during a child's early development can cause cognitive and motor impairment problems that can last throughout the child's lifetime. Breastfeeding an infant is an excellent choice, providing your baby with the most absorbable iron possible.

Iron is one of the few minerals for which unused amounts accumulate in your liver. Fortunately for women, excessive iron isn't too common. The main exception would be in older women, whose bodies simply don't need as much iron as they may be getting. While an iron deficiency can lead to serious health problems, excessive iron is just as bad, especially for men. Excess iron may encourage free radicals to damage cells. Excessive iron may increase your risk for cancer, primarily colon and liver cancers.

Excessive iron may also result in congestive heart failure. During and after a stroke, excessive iron may leak from the blood into the brain, worsening any damage caused by the stroke.

RECOMMENDED DIETARY ALLOWANCES
FOR IRON (MG)

AGE	RDA
Infants 0–6 mos	6
Infants 6 mos–1 year	10
Children 1–10 years	10
Men 11–18 years	5
Men 19–24 years	12
Men 25 years and older	15
Women 11–50 years	15
Women 51+ years	12
Pregnant Women	30
Breastfeeding Women	15

SOURCES OF IRON

Iron is one of the easier minerals to include in any diet. Iron is found in these foods:

- ▲ Organ meats, red meats
- ▲ Dried fruits
- ▲ Fruits, especially strawberries
- ▲ Cooked dried beans, lentils, and peas
- ▲ Dark green leafy vegetables
- ▲ Eggs
- ▲ Whole grains
- ▲ Pumpkin seeds
- ▲ Seaweed
- ▲ Green peas
- ▲ Tomato juice

▲ Nuts

▲ Broccoli

There are other methods for obtaining additional iron. One is to use an iron-clad cooking pot. Another is to cook foods in a minimum of water and not to overcook your food, as iron leaks out during the cooking process.

SUPPLEMENTS

Most men don't need iron supplements, unless recommended by your health care provider. Many women, however, would benefit from an iron supplement. You may choose to take it as a separate supplement, or as an added ingredient in a multivitamin pill. High-dose supplements, usually considered to be 30 mg or more, have been associated with side effects of nausea, constipation, and diarrhea.

CAUTIONS

Men should not take additional iron unless you have been advised to by your health care provider, or if you are a vegetarian or anemic. Another reminder to men: Do not take a multivitamin formulated for women—they almost always contain more iron since women generally need more iron than men.

Vitamin E may also reduce the effects of excessive iron.

Despite child-resistant caps and packaging currently being used, accidental iron overdose is the leading cause of poisoning deaths in children under the age of 6. Make sure you store any product containing iron out of the reach of any children.

MAGNESIUM

Magnesium is one of the macrominerals found in your body. More than one-half of your body's magnesium is located in your bones. One-quarter is in your muscles. The remainder is in your body fluids and soft tissues, including in the heart and kidneys. Magnesium is stored in your bones—an insurance policy to keep a good supply to the rest of the body when your magnesium intake is low.

MAGNESIUM'S ROLE IN YOUR BODY

Magnesium plays important roles in approximately three hundred functions in your body. Magnesium helps convert your food—the carbohydrates, fats, and proteins—into energy. It acts as a muscle relaxant. It helps the nerves transmit signals. It removes excessive toxic materials, such as ammonia, from your body. It protects you from heart disease by reducing the accumulation of cholesterol. High magnesium levels may even help you survive a heart attack. Many women report that magnesium relieves PMS symptoms. It also may be beneficial to migraine sufferers—it can prevent or reduce the duration of these extremely painful headaches.

Magnesium works along with calcium in many functions, and ideally their levels should be in balance. Calcium stimulates your muscles, while magnesium relaxes them. Calcium gives bones their strength. Magnesium gives them their elasticity.

Low magnesium levels and magnesium deficiencies are caused by other factors—not just diet. Excessive vomiting, diarrhea, kidney disease, long-term diuretic usage, alcohol abuse, and diabetes—all may contribute to lower levels of magnesium. Some antibiotics, laxatives, oral contraceptives, and chemotherapy drugs can also cause magnesium levels to drop. A low magnesium level affects all of the body's tissues, especially the heart, nerves, and kidneys. Heart failure can be caused by low magnesium, resulting from a magnesium-induced irregular heartbeat.

Symptoms of a magnesium deficiency are the following:

- ▲ Loss of appetite
- ▲ Muscle spasms
- ▲ Nausea
- ▲ Convulsions
- ▲ Depression
- ▲ Confusion
- ▲ Gastrointestinal disorders

Advanced magnesium deficiency is noted by hair loss, artery damage, and swollen gums. Magnesium deficiency can cause other serious health problems including diabetes, enlarged joints, lameness, and reproductive failure.

RECOMMENDED DIETARY ALLOWANCES FOR MAGNESIUM (MG)

AGE	RDA
Infants 0–6 mos	40
Infants 6 mos–1 year	60
Children 1–3 years	80
Children 4–6 years	120
Children 7–10 years	170
Men 11–14 years	270
Men 15–18 years	400
Men 19+ years	350
Women 11–14 years	280
Women 15–18 years	300
Women 19+ years	280
Pregnant Women	320
Breastfeeding Women (first 6 months)	355
Breastfeeding Women (second 6 months)	340

SOURCES OF MAGNESIUM

Dietary magnesium intakes are difficult to account for since very little magnesium is found in most common foods. Magnesium can be found in these foods:

- ▲ Almonds
- ▲ Beans
- ▲ Green vegetables
- ▲ Milk
- ▲ Molasses
- ▲ Pistachio nuts
- ▲ Some seafood
- ▲ Sunflower seeds
- ▲ Whole-grain breads and cereals

SUPPLEMENTS

Magnesium supplements are often recommended because of the lack of magnesium found in most diets. Magnesium is also required by the body for the proper function of B vitamins, especially B_1. Most experts recommend a supplement of less than 600 mg. Levels greater than that may cause loose stools.

CAUTIONS

Unless you have reduced kidney functions, your kidneys should be able to excrete any excessive amounts of magnesium you intake.

MANGANESE

Manganese is one micromineral about which not much is currently known compared to the other minerals in your body. It is thought that manganese can be readily replaced in its functions by magnesium.

MANGANESE'S ROLE IN YOUR BODY

Manganese may play a role in preventing osteoporosis, in that it contributes to healthy bones. It participates in the formation of connective tissues such as ligaments and tendons. Manganese is also needed for the digestion of proteins. Manganese may help lower sugar levels in diabetics who don't respond well to insulin.

In 1972, the first manganese deficiency was reported. Very few have been reported since that time. However, it is known that a manganese deficiency causes growth retardation, birth defects, bone malformations, seizures, general weakness, and impaired fertility.

RECOMMENDED DIETARY ALLOWANCES FOR MANGANESE

Currently there are no RDAs for manganese. There is little information about how much is needed, but an average intake should probably be at least from 2 mg to 9 mg per day.

SOURCES OF MANGANESE

Manganese is found in the following foods:

- ▲ Avocados
- ▲ Bananas
- ▲ Blueberries
- ▲ Chestnuts
- ▲ Coconuts
- ▲ Dried fruits
- ▲ Grapefruit
- ▲ Hazelnuts
- ▲ Milk
- ▲ Pineapple
- ▲ Raisins
- ▲ Spinach
- ▲ Sunflower seeds
- ▲ Whole-grain breads and cereals

SUPPLEMENTS

Manganese generally comes in high enough amounts in a multivitamin/multimineral supplement.

CAUTIONS

Excessive amounts of manganese may interfere with iron absorption.

MOLYBDENUM

Molybdenum is an essential micromineral found in the human body. It is found in all tissues, though it is primarily located in the bones, kidney, liver, and skin. Molybdenum is necessary for normal growth and development.

MOLYBDENUM'S ROLE IN YOUR BODY

Molybdenum plays several important roles in your body—pretty amazing for a mineral you have probably never heard about. One of its most important roles is to help release stored iron whenever necessary. It helps in the breakdown of nitrogen. Molybdenum assists cells in their functions. Molybdenum, along with vitamin B_2, helps convert food to energy. Molybdenum has been shown to be help prevent stomach and esophagus cancer.

Molybdenum deficiency is sometimes caused by lower levels of molybdenum in the soil where food is grown. The processing and refining of foods also eliminates molybdenum from many modern diets. A molybdenum deficiency may cause anemia, cancer, weight loss, and mouth and gum diseases. In older men, a molybdenum deficiency may cause impotence.

RECOMMENDED DIETARY ALLOWANCES FOR MOLYBDENUM

There are no RDAs for molybdenum. Some evidence indicates that an adult should receive between 75 and 250 mcg per day.

SOURCES FOR MOLYBDENUM

Molybdenum can be found in beans, dark green leafy vegetables, and peas.

SUPPLEMENTS

If larger doses are needed than what is available through diet or multivitamin/multimineral supplementation, it is available in injectable form through your health care provider.

CAUTIONS

Excess molybdenum may cause joint pain, stomach pain, and lower back pain. It may also cause your feet and lower legs to swell. Sufferers of liver or kidney disease may have elevated molybdenum levels.

PHOSPHORUS

Phosphorus is another one of the macrominerals found in your body. It is the second most abundant mineral in your body—only calcium has a greater presence. Eighty percent of the phosphorus in your body can be found in your bones and teeth. The remaining twenty percent is distributed among all of your cells.

PHOSPHORUS' ROLE IN YOUR BODY

Phosphorus, residing in all of your cells, can be found in all of the soft tissues of your body, such as your heart, kidneys, brain, and muscles. It is required for growth and maintenance of all of your body's tissues. Phosphorus is also needed for the conversion of the carbohydrates, fats, and proteins in your diet into energy. It also helps activate all of the B vitamins, allowing them to do their job. Phosphorus is needed to help provide strength and structure to your bones and teeth.

A phosphorus deficiency is extremely rare, although long-term or excessive use of antacids or anticonvulsant medications containing aluminum hydroxide can reduce the amount of phosphorus your body can absorb. Phosphorus deficiency can lead to tissue, nerve, muscles, and organ damage if allowed to go unchecked.

Overconsumption of phosphorus is more common, especially if you consume a high amount of convenience foods, soft drinks, and meat. A high phosphorus intake may lead to osteoporosis—by upsetting the fragile balance of calcium and phosphorus, not allowing the normal bone maintenance to occur.

RECOMMENDED DIETARY ALLOWANCES
FOR PHOSPHORUS (MG)

AGE	RDA
Infants 0–6 mos	300
Infants 6 mos–1 year	500
Children 1–10 years	800
Men and Women 11–24 years	1200
Men and Women 25+ years	800
Pregnant and Breastfeeding Women	1200

SOURCES OF PHOSPHORUS

Phosphorus is found in many protein-rich foods including the following:

- ▲ Meat, especially organ meats
- ▲ Fish
- ▲ Poultry
- ▲ Eggs
- ▲ Milk
- ▲ Whole-grain breads and cereals
- ▲ Peanut butter
- ▲ Oranges
- ▲ Bananas
- ▲ Cooked carrots
- ▲ Broccoli
- ▲ Beans
- ▲ Sunflower seeds

As noted previously, it is also found in many convenience foods and soft drinks; however, it is not recommended that you use these products to obtain phosphorus, since they make it difficult to maintain a healthy body due to high fat or sugar content.

SUPPLEMENTS

Most people probably would not benefit from a phosphorus supplement, since this mineral is so widely available in regular diets. However, some people may develop a deficiency, usually from prolonged use of antacids or anticonvulsant medications. Daily recommendations for supplementation is between 800 and 1,200 mg of phosphorus.

POTASSIUM

Potassium in another macromineral found in your body. Potassium is a major component of all the cells in your body.

POTASSIUM'S ROLE IN YOUR BODY

Potassium helps regulate the electrical charges within your body, controlling functions ranging from moving your legs to your heartbeat. Potassium is involved in muscle contraction, nerve conduction, heart functions, and energy production. It aids in lowering blood pressure, in part, by deactivating sodium before it raises blood pressure. Potassium may even be able to prevent you from developing high blood pressure in the first place.

African-Americans, who are at greater risk for developing high blood pressure, may especially want to monitor their potassium intake. People who take diuretics (water pills) may also benefit from increasing potassium. Potassium may be flushed out in urine when using diuretics. Laxative users may also need to add extra potassium. Laxatives, like diuretics, flush out needed nutrients. If you are easily fatigued, have general weakness, and muscle aches—you may be potassium deficient. Death can even occur if a potassium deficiency is left untreated for too long.

RECOMMENDED DIETARY ALLOWANCES FOR POTASSIUM

There are no RDAs for potassium.

SOURCES OF POTASSIUM

- ▲ Brewer's and torula yeast
- ▲ Fresh fruit, especially bananas
- ▲ Kelp and sea salt
- ▲ Milk
- ▲ Molasses
- ▲ Lean meats
- ▲ Parsley
- ▲ Peas
- ▲ Vegetables

SUPPLEMENTS

Potassium supplements should be considered if you are a diuretic or laxative user, or suffer from high blood pressure.

CAUTIONS

Potassium supplementation may be dangerous to those with impaired kidney function and to people on some forms of blood pressure—reducing medications. If you find yourself in one of these categories, ask your health care provider for more information before taking a potassium supplement.

SELENIUM

Selenium is a micromineral that is really finding itself in the news these days. Recent studies have affirmed that it may be beneficial in warding off cancer. But selenium was actually first discovered way back in 1817. It is named after the Greek word *selene*, which means "moon." However, it wasn't named as an essential mineral until the 1960s. Selenium is a mineral usually found in the soil where crops are grown. However, there are whole areas that have no or very little selenium in the soil, including China, Finland, and Sweden.

SELENIUM'S ROLE IN YOUR BODY

Cardiomyopathy, or heart weakness, can lead to death if the patient doesn't receive selenium supplements. Selenium helps the body produce antibodies to help keep the heart healthy. Selenium also acts as an antioxidant, preventing the formation of free radicals, which can damage the immune system. Where selenium levels are low in the soil, a higher rate of residents developing cancer has been noted.

High levels of dietary fat coupled with low levels of selenium may lead to breast and colon cancers. Selenium also guards against epithelial cancer—which is cancer of the membranes of the mouth, stomach, and lungs—esophageal cancer, prostate cancer, ovarian cancer, pancreas cancer, and skin cancer. Some researchers also believe selenium helps to stimulate the immune system. There is also reason to believe that it helps protect you from developing leukemia.

Selenium is also used in many shampoos to help control dandruff. It also may help with skin conditions, including acne. Selenium also helps reduce the inflammation of rheumatoid arthritis. Selenium helps to detoxify your body, ridding it of heavy metals that may suppress your immune system.

Sufferers of fibrocystic breast disease, which causes painful breast lumps, may find some relief with selenium. Selenium is also known for improving moods, while reducing anxiety, depression, and fatigue.

A selenium deficiency can cause rheumatoid arthritis in young children or adults. It may even occur if the mother was selenium-deficient during pregnancy. Since selenium and vitamin E both work together to make antibodies that protect the liver, a deficiency can cause liver degeneration. Liver disease is also more common in people with a lower selenium level. A deficiency may also cause heart disease—often prematurely.

Symptoms of a selenium deficiency include anemia, muscle weakness, muscle soreness, and damage to your pancreas.

RECOMMENDED DIETARY ALLOWANCES
FOR SELENIUM (MCG)

AGE	RDA
Infants 0–6 mos	10
Infants 6 mos–1 year	15
Children 1–3 years	20
Children 4–6 years	20
Children 7–10 years	30
Men 11–14 years	40
Men 15–18 years	50
Men 19+ years	70
Women 11–14 years	45
Women 15–18 years	50
Women 19+ years	55
Pregnant Women	65
Breastfeeding Women	75

SOURCES OF SELENIUM

To add more selenium to your food plan, try these foods:

▲ Whole wheat grains

▲ Brown rice

▲ Poultry

▲ Broccoli and cabbage

▲ Brazil nuts

▲ Clove garlic

▲ Mushrooms

▲ Seafood

▲ Dairy products

▲ Organ meats and lean meats

Selenium is also found in lesser amounts in other fruits and vegetables.

SUPPLEMENTS

Too much selenium is toxic, stimulating some forms of cancer. Symptoms of toxicity to watch out for include garlic breath, nervousness, loose fingernails, loose hair, vomiting, and fatigue.

CAUTIONS

It is wisest to never take a selenium supplement over 200 mcg, especially when adding more selenium-rich foods to your daily diet.

SODIUM

Sodium is another macromineral you may be surprised to learn your body actually does need. So often you are bombarded with information warning you not to use too much sodium. The reality is, that sodium is just as necessary as any other mineral. In fact, you can't live without it!

SODIUM'S ROLE IN YOUR BODY

Sodium is essential to proper nerve, muscle, and stomach functions. It also keeps cell walls penetrable so they can be properly maintained. Sodium also regulates the amount of water in your body.

For many years it has been thought that too much sodium raised blood pressure. However, there is no current consensus on this topic. Some studies have shown that a low sodium level in a person with high blood pressure may increase their risk for heart attack.

Signs of sodium deficiency are confusion, dehydration, lowered blood sugar levels, weakness, and heart palpitations. Since sodium can be found in almost everything we consume today, sodium deficiency has become rare, although still possible.

RECOMMENDED DIETARY ALLOWANCES FOR SODIUM

There are no RDAs for sodium. Most experts recommend that you have no more than about 2000 mg of sodium per day.

SOURCES OF SODIUM

- ▲ Bread and cereal
- ▲ Canned soups
- ▲ Cheese
- ▲ Meat
- ▲ Pickled foods
- ▲ Potato chips
- ▲ Salad dressings
- ▲ Shellfish

SUPPLEMENTS

Sometimes sodium is used to treat dehydration. Although some experts feel one can safely consume 5,000 mg of sodium, most concur that 2,000 mg is adequate. 2,000 mg of sodium is equal to one teaspoon.

CAUTIONS

Excess sodium may cause edema (caused by excessive fluid build-up in cells.) It may also cause or worsen high blood pressure. Excessive sodium also can cause a potassium deficiency. Untreated, high sodium levels may lead to heart, liver, or kidney disease.

ZINC

Zinc is another important micromineral. Most people don't currently get enough zinc. In fact, it is estimated that one-half of older people get less than two-thirds of the RDA amount of zinc in their daily food intake. There are many reasons for these low amount of zinc in our diets today:

- ▲ Dietary fiber inhibits zinc absorption
- ▲ Including less red meats in your diet may cause zinc deficiency
- ▲ Aging—if you are past 50, your body automatically absorbs less zinc
- ▲ Vegetarian diet interferes with zinc absorption
- ▲ Calorie-restricted diet limits your ability to take in enough zinc

ZINC'S ROLE IN YOUR BODY

Zinc is essential to many body functions. One of the most important functions for men is that zinc promotes fertility. Zinc plays an important role in the production of testosterone, which is the main male hormone. A low zinc level in a man's body creates a low level of testosterone. A low amount of testosterone makes for fewer sperm. And the sperm you have show signs of decreased motility—that's the ability of sperm to wiggle around, eventually making its way through the female's reproductive system, looking for an egg to fertilize. So men, if you and your partner are trying to conceive and have been unsuccessful, have your zinc levels checked!

Amazing as it is, that's not all that zinc can do for you. Zinc also helps protect your vision. Zinc helps regulate your insulin levels. By creating new skin, zinc helps heal wounds. By helping to produce new cells, zinc keeps your immune system healthy and functioning when you need it.

One of the most recent discoveries has been that zinc, especially when taken in the form of a lozenge, helps prevent symptoms associated with colds. If you already have a cold, taking zinc at the first sign of one may help shorten the length of the cold. Be advised, though, that most of the zinc lozenges currently on the market do cause some stomach upset or discomfort.

It would take 2,400 calories per day for you to get enough zinc in your diet naturally. Most women would find themselves overweight consuming those kinds of calories. Add to this the fact that many people have cut down on meats and increased their fiber intakes, it's no wonder that many people are zinc deficient.

Zinc deficiency causes many varied symptoms and some results can be devastating. Acne, eczema, hair loss, decreased sense of taste and smell, and the absence of menstrual periods are all symptoms of zinc deficiency. Some of the end results of a zinc deficiency include:

▲ Nerve damage

▲ Depression

▲ Birth defects

▲ Delayed fetal development

Low zinc levels in adolescents can also stunt bone growth and may lead to the development of osteoporosis later in life.

RECOMMENDED DIETARY ALLOWANCES FOR ZINC (MG)

AGE	RDA
Infants	5
Children 1–10 years	5
Men 11+ years	15
Women 11+ years	12
Pregnant Women	15
Breastfeeding Women (first 6 months)	19
Breastfeeding Women (second 6 months)	16

SOURCES OF ZINC

Zinc can be found in some of the foods you consume. However, since so many people are vegetarians and many others have also increased their fiber intakes, zinc deficiency is becoming increasingly common. It should be noted that thirty percent of the total population is thought to be deficient in zinc. Foods containing good amounts of zinc include:

- ▲ Seafood, especially oysters
- ▲ Meat
- ▲ Beans
- ▲ Nuts
- ▲ Whole grains
- ▲ Fortified cereals
- ▲ Sesame seeds

SUPPLEMENTATS

Zinc supplementation is an excellent idea for many people. The difficult part may be to take enough zinc, but not too much. High levels of zinc can cause problems, too. If you wish to try more than the RDA, you may be wise to first consult with your health care provider. Zinc needs to be always taken with food or you may experience stomach irritation. Taking 1,500 mg or more of calcium daily interferes with zinc absorption. In this case, it would be advisable to increase your zinc intake by another 10 mg per day.

CAUTIONS

Zinc toxicity symptoms are nausea, metallic taste in mouth, cramps, vomiting, dizziness, and chills.

A high zinc level may actually suppress your immune system and inhibit copper absorption.

CHAPTER 4

Other Nonherbal Supplements

Dietary supplements have been around for years. There is nothing new about humans trying to live longer, healthier lives—using whatever means available to accomplish that goal. But this nonherbal supplement category is where things can get a little bit tricky. You know what vitamins and minerals are. The world of nonherbal supplements is much more vague—and often confusing.

The word supplement itself means to complete or to make whole. How do you figure out what is needed to make you whole? Does your health care provider believe in supplements? How can you decipher the truth from the hype about various supplements? This chapter provides general information about the role of nonherbal supplements in maintaining health. We then give information about specific supplements, including enzymes, amino acids, and other dietary supplements. It is beyond the scope of this book to discuss the thousands of herbal supplements on the market.

WHO NEEDS NONHERBAL SUPPLEMENTS

There are many reasons why you may choose to take a supplement. Many of us are continuously trying to lose just a few pounds—or more. Constant dieting can leave you with a low-fat, high-fiber diet that is generally good for you. But one drawback of this diet is that some necessary ingredients for your good health—such as amino acids—are often found more concentrated in the high-fat foods you're probably avoiding. And eating a diet rich in fiber—again for the most part very good for your overall health—may cause elimination or flushing out of many nutrients before they can be utilized by your body.

You may also want to consider supplementation if:

- ▲ You have impaired absorption of nutrients.
- ▲ You have an infection.
- ▲ You are 55 years old or older. Older people often do not eat enough and are not able to absorb as many nutrients from the food they do eat. If you are older, you may benefit most from supplements that increase brain functions, including memory.
- ▲ You use medications such as diuretics (water pills) or street drugs that inhibit absorption of nutrients.
- ▲ You are under heavy stress.
- ▲ You are suffering major trauma.
- ▲ You are a heavy user of alcohol. Using alcohol inhibits and damages your liver—upsetting the operations of the whole body.
- ▲ You eat a vegetarian diet, especially if you are a vegan (eat no food from animals, including dairy products and eggs). Vegetarians, and especially vegans, rarely consume enough substances naturally since many needed substances are found primarily in meat or dairy products. Vegetarians, even vegans, can still take supplements—there are forms manufactured from plants or through a chemical process that contain no animal products.

SUPPLEMENT SAFETY

The FDA defines dietary supplements as any product you take by mouth. Other than vitamins and minerals, dietary supplements currently on store shelves include amino acids, enzymes, extracts, metabolites, hormones, organ tissues, and herbal preparations. The FDA does not regulate the sale or manufacture of dietary supplements, although they do have some rules, primarily regarding the labeling of supplements. The label must follow these guidelines:

- ▲ Be truthful.
- ▲ Clearly state what the dietary ingredient is.
- ▲ Tell you what other ingredients are contained in the

supplement, which are normally sugar, starch, or preservatives.

▲ Contain enough information about the product for you to make an educated decision about purchasing the supplement.

Generally, the FDA relies on the manufacturers of supplements to make sure the ingredients are safe and reliable. However, if you or your health care provider suspect that a dietary supplement has made you ill or caused a serious side effect, you should contact the FDA to register your information. The FDA's MedWatch hotline is 1-800-FDA-1088 and their Website is located at is http://www.fda.gov/medwatch/report/consumer/consumer.htm.

There has been at least one occasion when the FDA stepped in and made a product unavailable in the United States. In 1989, there was an outbreak of eosinophilia-myalgia syndrome (**EMS**), causing at least 1,500 illnesses and 38 deaths. This outbreak was traced to a dietary supplement, L-trytophan, which was commonly used to aid insomniacs. It was due to the contamination of the product coming from one manufacturer located in Japan. But even though there were other manufacturers of L-tryptophan whose products caused no known problems, this supplement is still banned for sale in the United States.

The sad truth is that the FDA generally waits until there is a public health emergency to take any action. Currently, there are many reported serious health complications, including death, with ephedrine, a chemical found in many herbal supplements. The FDA has issued an advisory about ephedrine, but has taken no further action.

COMMON FORMS OF SUPPLEMENTS

Supplements come in many forms, including the following:

▲ Capsules
▲ Liquids

- Pills
- Powders
- Tablets

If a high concentration is needed, some supplements are much more reasonably priced if purchased in powdered form. Many of the powders available are odorless and tasteless, blending very nicely into applesauce or pudding. If you have difficulty swallowing a large uncoated tablet, especially if it is round, a capsule, liquid, or powder may be the best choice.

Some supplement tablets and capsules may not dissolve quickly enough to be of much benefit. If you prefer a capsule or tablet instead of a powder, try dropping one into a glass of water—then watch to see if it dissolves within a few minutes. If it doesn't, your body probably won't be able to dissolve it quickly enough to be of much benefit either. In this case, try a different brand or try a powder or liquid form of the supplement.

CATEGORIES OF SUPPLEMENTS

This chapter will deal with supplements in various categories including enzymes, amino acids, fatty acids, and hormones. We'll give details about uses and dosages recommended by some nutrition experts, when available. This is for your information only, and is not intended to be prescriptive. There are no formal RDAs for these types of supplements. Before using these types of nutritional supplements, we recommend that you talk with a qualified health care provider.

Many people benefit from the use of these supplements, some of which are difficult to obtain through your daily food intake. Some of these nutrients are required for your body to manufacture other products for healthy living and disease prevention. Some even may help your body reverse some of the damage caused by diseases like high blood pressure.

ENZYMES

Enzymes are special proteins that aid the various chemical reactions within your body, a process called catalysis. Vitamins are the most well-known types of enzymes. In addition, other chemicals also act as enzymes to aid body processes. Some of these are available in supplemental form or by prescription.

COENZYME Q-10

One of the most exciting supplements on the market today is coenzyme Q-10. Q-10 is a combination of ubiquinone, which is used by your cells to burn energy, and vitamin Q. Japan, Europe, Israel, Sweden, and Denmark all are countries that have been using this product since its discovery in beef heart mitochondria in 1957. Many folks in these countries take Q-10 as a preventative supplement; however, Q-10 also is used for disease control—primarily for congestive heart failure, a slow, degenerative disease in which the heart muscle gradually loses its ability to contract. The benefits of Q-10 have long been realized by other countries; now it is a common supplement in the United States.

Q-10 is produced by your body and is vitally needed for good health. Q-10 is primarily stored in the kidneys, liver, and, of course, the heart. Production amounts begin to decline around age twenty. By middle age, you may find yourself deficient in Q-10. Many of those over age fifty with degenerative heart disease have been found to be lacking in Q-10 levels.

It is suspected that low levels of Q-10 means that your body doesn't absorb enough vitamins, namely folate, niacin, vitamin B_6, vitamin B_{12}, and vitamin C. These vitamins are necessary for your body to convert amino acids into tyrosine, another amino acid. Tyrosine is needed for the production of Q-10.

Primarily, Q-10's function is to help with the prevention and improvement of congestive heart failure. It has been noted that the level of Q-10 in a diseased heart is much lower than in a healthy heart. After taking Q-10 supplements, some people needing heart transplants have been able to take their names off the list due to their dramatic improvement. Others have been able to stay alive awaiting their transplant through their usage of Q-10. In studies done in Japan, approximately seventy percent of patients having congestive heart failure obtained positive clinical benefits. Heart disease patients in general are able to live longer, leading more active and healthier lives through their use of Q-10. Their improvement is often said to be very clear and dramatic.

Q-10 also may reduce blood pressure. One study showed that approximately fifty percent of the participants with high blood pressure were able to reduce the amount of medications used to treat it. Another twenty-five percent were able to control their hypertension by only using Q-10. Q-10 achieves this through the cleansing and strengthening of the arteries.

Q-10 is known for its ability to protect the mitochondria in cells. The mitochondria, among other activities, help convert food to usable energy. This may also help prevent degenerative brain disease, such as Alzheimer's Disease and Lou Gehrig's disease, by protecting the mitochondria in brain cells. Even gradual memory loss and loss of normal brain function may be prevented with an adequate supply of Q-10.

Q-10 has other jobs, as well:

- ▲ Purifying the liver
- ▲ Preventing chronic obstructive pulmonary disease (**COPD**)
- ▲ Boosting your immune system
- ▲ Preventing cancer from developing through its ability to ward off cell damage by free radicals
- ▲ Relieving symptoms associated with cancer chemotherapy
- ▲ Reducing damage to normal tissue from chemotherapy treatments

One of the ways Q-10 is created naturally is through vigorous exercise. You can also get one day's supply by eating a pound of sardines! But vigorous exercise or the consumption of huge amounts of sardines would be necessary almost each and every day. Supplementing, in this case, is really the only way to obtain greater amounts of this vital enzyme. Q-10 is not generally found in a multivitamin/multimineral supplement, but must be purchased and taken separately.

Unfortunately, Q-10 is often more expensive than other supplements—though its benefits are certainly many. Q-10 also takes time to work—don't expect to see results overnight. Results aren't felt until at least four weeks, even up to three months, after beginning a Q-10 regimen. Fortunately, there are no known side effects from taking Q-10 supplements.

If you are in generally good health, many nutrition experts recommend taking 30 mg of Q-10 daily. If you have a chronic disease, other than heart disease, or are at risk for developing a chronic disease, take 50–150 mg every day. Heart patients are often instructed to take 120 mg twice daily. Remember, too, do not reduce or stop prescription medications without letting your health care provider know.

DIGESTIVE ENZYMES

Certain supplements contain enzymes intended to aid digestion. These enzymes usually come combined with other enzymes or are contained in multivitamin supplements in various combinations. Some of the digestive enzymes available include the following:

- ▲ Pepsin
- ▲ Papain
- ▲ Betaine hydrochloride
- ▲ Pancreatin
- ▲ Bromolin

Other enzymes break down specific foods:

- ▲ Lactase helps break down milk products. It is available in tablets or powder.
- ▲ Protease aids in the digestion of protein. It is available in supplemental form.

Many other enzymes, such as lipase, work on specific foods. However, these enzymes are usually found only in multi-enzyme supplements.

AMINO ACIDS

Amino acids are usually known as the building blocks of protein. It's easy to see why that analogy is so often used—amino acids are assembled together in various combinations to make proteins. Without protein, we cannot sustain life. Therefore, without amino acids to create the protein, we can't live. Protein is essential for growth and development. Protein is also used to manufacture hormones, enzymes, and tissues.

Amino acids work together with vitamins and minerals to do their jobs. Taking vitamin B_6 or vitamin C with amino acids helps your body absorb the amino acids better. If you are using amino acid supplementation to treat an illness or injury, it is advisable to take them on an empty stomach. This way, they are not having to compete with the vitamins, minerals, and other amino acids in your food.

There are two basic categories of amino acids: essential amino acids and nonessential amino acids. The word "essential" in this phrase can be misleading. It doesn't imply that the essential amino acids are more important than the nonessential amino acids. It actually means that the essential amino acids are not able to be manufactured by your body. They must be taken on a daily basis through your diet or through supplementation.

Your body is a busy little factory. It takes the essential amino acids that you put into your body and make the nonessential amino acids out of the essential amino acids as they are needed. Then it takes all of the amino acids and makes lots of other products out of them—including protein. Amino acids all need to cooperate and work together. A deficiency in even one amino acid can disrupt this whole process.

This process of making other amino acids is called synthesis and goes on continually in your body. Some amino acids act as carriers—and even have the ability to cross over the blood–brain barrier. The blood–brain barrier is a defensive shield around the brain in order to protect it from toxins. This barrier can also make it difficult for needed materials to get across the barrier. Fortunately, amino acids are able to cross this barrier.

> ## SELECTING AMINO ACIDS
> *Amino acid supplements are often sold in groups—you may find a supplement containing two or more amino acids in it. They are usually grouped in specific combinations to achieve specific results, such as to provide more energy. Some amino acids are also sold as single supplements.*

ESSENTIAL AMINO ACIDS

Essential amino acids are called "essential" simply because they must be taken in to your body through food or supplements. Your body cannot make any more as needed, like it does the nonessential amino acids. It takes the essential amino acids that you have taken in and synthesizes them into whatever nonessential amino acids it requires. Unfortunately for those attempting to get essential amino acids in their diet, they are most often found in foods high in fat—such as meats, cheese, or eggs. This has made supplementation very attractive to many people.

The eight essential amino acids include:

▲ Isoleucine

▲ Leucine

▲ Lysine

▲ Methionine

▲ Phenylalanine

▲ Threonine

▲ Tryptophan

▲ Valine

Essential amino acids are required for your body to manufacture proteins and nonessential amino acids, but other than that, their functions remain a bit of a mystery. More information is known about the nonessential amino acids. One of the primary things we do know about essential amino acids, however, is that they are absolutely necessary to maintain a healthy body.

ISOLEUCINE

Isoleucine is thought to help regulate blood sugar levels. It also helps to regulate energy levels. Athletes have long known the value of isoleucine—they believe it increases their energy and endurance levels.

Some physicians have used isoleucine to treat side effects caused by the treatment of Maple Syrup Urine Disease (**MSUD**). MSUD is an inherited disease, characterized by the urine smelling like maple syrup. Treatment of infants with this condition often includes the use of an amino acid-free formula, which causes skin lesions and diarrhea. It was noted that by adding isoleucine to the formula, lesions and diarrhea disappeared.

More recently, isoleucine has been used in combination with AZT, a drug used to treat patients infected with HIV, the virus that causes AIDS. The new product, IAZT, has been found to be more effective than AZT alone. IAZT is better absorbed into the cells and is less toxic to cells than AZT.

Isoleucine is able to penetrate the blood–brain barrier. Isoleucine is highly soluble, enabling it to help transport other medications over this barrier to treat HIV infection of the nervous system.

It is often difficult to tell what a deficiency of an essential amino acid would cause, since any given amino acid is used by the body in so many ways. But it is known that a deficiency of isoleucine does cause similar symptoms of hypoglycemia (low blood sugar), which deprives your muscles and cells of energy that is provided by glucose. These symptoms include:

- ▲ Dizziness
- ▲ Weakness
- ▲ Trembling
- ▲ Blurred vision and speech
- ▲ Headache
- ▲ Tingling in the hands or lips

An isoleucine deficiency has often been found in studies of people with various mental disorders. Research continues to see if there is a true connection between isoleucine deficiency and mental disorders.

LEUCINE

Many positive effects are derived from leucine. Leucine is essential for the growth and development of children. This is due to the ability leucine has to increase production of the growth hormone. As infants and children grow, their bodies need and use more growth hormone than as we need as adults. Higher leucine levels means higher levels of growth hormone—enabling the baby to grow and development as much as required.

In conjunction with valine and isoleucine, two other essential amino acids, leucine helps protect and provide energy to your muscles.

Some surgeons have found that leucine is helpful for use with their surgical patients, because of its ability to promote the healing of bones, muscle tissues, and skin.

Leucine also may help lower blood sugar levels in those who have moderately high levels.

Studies of elderly men have found that their livers excrete high levels of leucine during meals. This could lead to a lower availability of leucine available to the body and may require an increase in leucine intakes to make up for this additional excretion.

LYSINE

Lysine is one of the better known amino acids. Lysine has many attributes—one of the best known is its ability to prevent or shorten the duration of cold sores. However, lysine is known to do much more than that.

Lysine also helps your body absorb calcium by reducing the loss of calcium through urination. Lysine plays a role in the formation of bone, cartilage, and connective tissues (tendons and ligaments). Lysine is an important antioxidant that attacks free radicals, strengthening the immune system. Lysine is also needed for the production of the fibrous tissue called collagen, which develops into skin tissues.

Lysine may alleviate the symptoms of chronic fatigue syndrome. It is estimated that more than two million Americans, primarily women, suffer from this disease. Chronic fatigue syndrome is characterized by fatigue, a low-grade fever, sore throat, muscle aches, joint pain, and sleep disturbances. There have been reports of people with this disease finding relief through taking lysine supplements in higher amounts—2,000 mg per day.

Lysine relieves symptoms of the many different forms of the herpes virus. One form, herpes zoster, is more commonly known as shingles. It occurs as a result of a hidden chickenpox virus that resurfaces during times of great stress or when the immune system is weakened. Red, painful blisters may appear anywhere on your body during an outbreak. You also may have flu-like symptoms of chills, fever, nausea, or diarrhea. The taking of lysine is thought to both prevent future outbreaks and shorten the duration of a current outbreak.

It is estimated that as many as twenty million Americans are afflicted with genital herpes, otherwise known as herpes simplex II. Shortly after exposure, an afflicted person experiences flu-like symptoms: fever, chills, nausea, and diarrhea. Blister-like sores, on or near the genitals, buttocks, or inner thigh, appear approximately three weeks after exposure to the virus. The blisters are painful and may cause a burning sensation. Genital herpes is a risk especially to pregnant women. If there is an outbreak at the time of delivery, your doctor will probably recommend giving birth by Cesarean section to protect the newborn. Genital herpes is also thought to contribute to the development of cervical cancer in women.

Another form of herpes is herpes simplex I—otherwise known as cold sores or fever blisters. These painful blisters usually occur on the lips, but may also appear inside the mouth and usually take a week or more to disappear.

All forms of herpes lie dormant in the body until something stimulates it to break out. Herpes is a recurrent disease that requires you to control and manage it. Subsequent outbreaks of herpes are most often caused by:

▲ Colds or another infection

▲ Exposure to sunlight

- ▲ Upset stomach
- ▲ Stress
- ▲ Fatigue

Taking lysine at the first sign of an outbreak has been shown to shorten the duration of the outbreak. Many people take lysine on a daily basis to help prevent an outbreak of herpes.

Bell's palsy is a virus that causes facial paralysis—making one side of your face droopy. There are some studies showing that lysine aids in the recovery from this disease, which can otherwise take many months or even longer.

Meniere's disease is an inner ear disorder that can cause severe dizziness and hearing loss. Studies show lysine helping people suffering from this disease.

Some physicians have found that lysine helps patients recover from sports injuries. This is probably due to the fact that lysine helps build muscle proteins, which can speed recovery.

Some studies that show lysine—along with the amino acid arginine—when given to young adults increased their secretion of growth hormone. Some believe that this discovery may help researchers find methods to delay the aging process, since we naturally secrete lower levels of growth hormone as we age.

Low levels of lysine have been found in patients suffering from Parkinson's disease, depression, asthma, and kidney disease. The link between these diseases and lysine isn't currently known—but research is continuing.

A lysine deficiency has many symptoms:

- ▲ Lack of energy
- ▲ Poor appetite
- ▲ Weight loss
- ▲ Reproductive disorders
- ▲ Anemia
- ▲ Hair loss

Lysine is found in cottage cheese, wheat germ, and avocado. Supplements are also widely available in varying amounts.

METHIONINE

Methionine often joins with lysine to create carnitine, a nonessential amino acid that helps keep hearts healthy. Carnitine reduces the level of cholesterol and triglycerides in the bloodstream, helping to fight off atherosclerosis, while reducing the risk of a heart attack.

Methionine also works on its own to prevent heart problems. It helps with the breakdown of fats, helping to prevent a buildup of fat in your liver and arteries. A buildup of fat eventually may obstruct the blood flow through the arteries.

In patients with incontinence (loss of bladder control) and infants with diaper rash, methionine may be beneficial. It is used to make urine more acidic, controlling strong urine odors while relieving skin irritation.

Methionine is known to help protect against radiation. It also helps detoxify your body of heavy metals by synthesizing into cysteine, then into glutathion—which is a key neutralizer of toxins found in the liver.

Methionine has a relationship with schizophrenia. It has been noted that it reduces the levels of histamines. A high level of histamines is found in patients with schizophrenia and some health care providers are trying methionine supplementation with their schizophrenia patients.

A higher intake of methionine creates a higher level of methyl. A higher level of methyl reduces the risk of colorectal cancer—cancer of the colon or rectum.

Some less developed countries, where acetaminophen overdoses are common, have found a unique use for methionine. Acetaminophen is a commonly purchased over-the-counter pain reliever. Whether the overdose is accidental or not, liver damage—even to the point of death—often occurs. Researchers have discovered that methionine may prevent liver damage from an acetaminophen overdose. Some countries are even considering adding methionine to each acetaminophen tablet.

Meat, soybeans, and yogurt are a few of the food sources for methionine.

PHENYLALANINE

Phenylalanine is another one of the eight essential amino acids. If you look at some brands of artificial sweeteners, you will find it listed as an ingredient.

Phenylalanine synthesizes into tyrosine. Tyrosine is a nonessential amino acid that synthesizes into both dopamine and norepinephrine, both neurotransmitters involved in functions of the central nervous systems.

Phenylalanine, in this way, helps regulate moods, decreases pain, suppresses appetites, and may improve your memory and learning skills. It also helps to regulate heart rate, blood pressure, and blood sugar levels in blood.

Some health care providers are currently using phenylalanine to treat arthritis, menstrual cramps, and obesity. Some are testing phenylalanine to treat brain disorders as varied as depression, schizophrenia, and Parkinson's disease.

Current research indicates that phenylalanine may be useful to **HIV** (human immunodeficiency virus) infected patients. It appears to stop the coupling between the HIV infection and **T-cells,** which are a type of white blood cell that plays a part in the immune system.

In rare cases, a person may be born with a defective gene that controls the metabolism of phenylalanine. This may cause seizures or mental retardation.

It is suggested that you not supplement your intake of phenylalanine if you are pregnant, have diabetes, high blood pressure, or skin cancer.

THREONINE

Threonine is found in the central nervous system, heart, and skeletal muscles. Threonine helps maintain the proper balance of proteins in the body. It also is needed for the formation of collagen, which helps form bones, cartilage, tendons, and other connective tissues of the body.

Along with aspartic acid, a nonessential amino acid, threonine aids in liver and lipotropic functions, preventing an excessive buildup of fats to accumulate in the liver.

Threonine helps produce antibodies, which play a major role in the immune system by combating infection, bacteria, and toxins that make their way into the body. This is how threonine helps you to fight off illness.

Some researchers are finding threonine helps their patients battle amyotrophic lateral sclerosis (**ALS**), commonly referred to as Lou Gehrig's disease. ALS causes progressive muscular atrophy, or muscular wasting. Some studies indicate that within forty-eight hours of taking threonine, ALS patients report several improvements in their condition. This includes better voice control, decreased spasticity, increased energy, less drooling, and an easier time swallowing.

Threonine is found primarily in meats and other animal products. Threonine is present only in low amounts in grains. Because of this, many vegetarians, especially vegans, are deficient in this essential amino acid.

TRYPTOPHAN

Tryptophan is an essential amino acid that is no longer available over-the-counter. Tryptophan had been used by consumers for over twenty years as a treatment for insomnia, depression, premenstrual symptoms, and chronic pain.

Tryptophan works by affecting the brain chemistry. It converts to serotonin, which is a neurotransmitter that allows nerve cells to communicate. Serotonin helps regulate sleep, pain, appetite, and moods.

In 1989, trytophan was banned by the FDA. This occurrence happened as a result of thousands of users coming down with a rare blood and muscle disorder. This disorder resulted in thirty-eight deaths, and many afflicted with this disorder still suffer the effects. It was eventually linked to a Japanese manufacturer of tryptophan that introduced an impurity when it changed its manufacturing process.

Tryptophan is still available in foods—though not in high enough amounts to be therapeutic. Milk, spinach, and turkey all contain tryptophan.

VALINE

Another essential amino acid is valine. Used as a source of energy by muscles, it shouldn't be surprising that valine is found in highly concentrated amounts in muscle tissues. It actually acts like a stimulant—which can promote a feeling of well being while increasing vitality.

Valine also helps to correct the fragile balancing act of amino acids in situations that may throw them off-balance—such as going through drug withdrawal.

NONESSENTIAL AMINO ACIDS

Nonessential amino acids are certainly no less important than essential amino acids. It's just that your body can synthesize, or make, them out of the essential amino acids. In some ways, their job may be more important, but they can't exist without the presence of essential amino acids. Nonessential amino acids are also needed to build other amino acids and proteins. So they are just as important to life as essential amino acids.

Many of the nonessential amino acids are available in supplement form. They are sold in single supplements, combined with other amino acids, or even included in some multivitamin supplements.

ALANINE

One of the most important functions of alanine, a nonessential amino acid, is that of a diagnostic tool. Testing levels of alanine oftentimes alerts health care providers to the presence of liver disease—since many liver diseases cause a greater secretion of alanine.

Donated blood has been tested for various forms of viral hepatitis, including hepatitis C, by testing for levels of alanine in the blood. Hepatitis is an inflammation of the liver that may cause severe long-term symptoms including jaundice and abdominal pain.

Testing has shown higher levels of alanine in patients who are obese, or in patients who use drugs or alcohol excessively. There is also concern that drinking of unfiltered coffee may increase the alanine level. Currently, the level of alanine and these diseases have not shown if alanine affects the disease, or if the disease affects the alanine level, but research is always continuing.

If any test shows a higher than normal level of alanine in one's system, it is extremely important to follow through with a thorough medical evaluation, including taking a look at your medical history and lifestyle issues that may be affecting the alanine level. If no obvious cause is found, it would be advisable to re-do the test, just to double-check its accuracy. If the test shows high levels again, it would be a good idea to have your health care provider check for liver disease.

Alanine has also been shown to help in the metabolism of glucose—the process that provides you with energy.

Infants suffering from dehydration due to diarrhea, often are fed oral hydration therapy—a special solution that contains alanine. Alanine helps the infant's body absorb the water and sodium in the solution, replacing the water lost during through the diarrhea.

ARGININE

Another nonessential, though important, amino acid is arginine. Arginine has been known to help build up muscles, while decreasing body fat. It also helps release energy to muscles, through its ability to help in fat tissue catabolism. Catabolism is the process that breaks down the complex molecules into simpler ones, resulting in a release of energy.

Arginine helps promote a healthy heart by improving coronary blood flow. Arginine allows the blood vessels to dilate, or open, more—thus allowing blood to flow freely through them. It accomplishes this through the reversal of endothelial abnormalities. The endothelium is a thin layer of flat cells that line the blood vessels. If they are abnormal in size or shape, they don't allow blood to pass freely through the blood vessels. This has the added benefit of reducing blood pressure.

Impotence is a medical condition that, in some cases, may be caused by reduced blood flow to the penis. Arginine is found in seminal fluid. Many health care providers are using arginine as a tool to treat impotence.

A deficiency of arginine during the formative years may delay sexual maturity in young men. Studies have shown that when arginine is administered to young adult males, it causes an increase in secretion of growth hormone.

High levels of arginine have been found in skin and connective tissues. Arginine helps heal and repair damage done to tissues. Some also report relief from arthritis inflammation by increasing their intakes of arginine.

Another benefit of this amino acid is the use of arginine along with conventional cancer treatments, resulting in the reduction of breast tumors.

Arginine helps stimulate the pancreas to release insulin. This is why low levels of arginine have been found in patients suffering from insulinopenia—the failure to secrete insulin as needed.

Arginine can enhance the immune system, therefore, slowing the growth of tumors and cancers. It does this primarily through one of its products—argine deiminase—which destroys other amino acids that contribute to the growth of cancer cells.

Ongoing studies are have shown arginine to be beneficial to patients with AIDS. It can increase the health of the T-cells (white blood cells) by increasing their size and their activity levels.

By neutralizing ammonia stored in the liver, arginine may benefit those suffering from liver ailments due to cirrhosis, which results in an inflammation of the liver.

Surgeons have found further benefits to this amazing amino acid. After surgery, patients are often fed a liquid diet containing arginine combined with antibiotics. This forms a salt-free and stable solution that is soluble, or dissolvable, in water, which increases its effectiveness. This helps to rapidly restore an immune system by getting vital nutrients to it as quickly as possible, enabling a speedier recovery.

One word of caution—it is not advisable to take arginine supplements if you have a viral infection such as herpes, are pregnant or breast-feeding, or suffer from schizophrenia. Arginine may possibly have a negative effect on these conditions—in the case of viral infection, it is possible that arginine in too high amounts may promote the growth and spread of the virus.

ASPARTIC ACID

Aspartic acid is a nonessential acid that can be found in protein. Aspartic acid is known for its ability to increase stamina, decrease fatigue, and remove excessive ammonia from the body, which may increase from vigorous exercise.

D-aspartate, a derivative of aspartic acid, when combined with N-methyl, forms NMDA, activating other substances used in neurological development and function. NMDA helps alleviate impaired neurological functions such as learning and memory disorders, especially when stress related.

Aspartic acid helps produce immunoglobulins—immune system proteins that function as antibodies to combat infection by binding with specific antigens, rendering them useless.

Aspartic acid is used along with opiate medications such as morphine to relieve chronic pain. Opiate medications often decrease in effectiveness over time. Adding aspartic acid to the treatment maintains the opiate's effectiveness.

CARNITINE

Carnitine is a nonessential amino acid—it is formed by the essential amino acids lysine and methionine. Carnitine can also be found in meat, especially red meats, and dairy products. Commercial carnitine production is being increased by dramatic proportions, including by those manufacturers producing it for use in animal feed.

One of the most important functions of carnitine is its ability to help stimulate the brain. It accomplishes this feat by helping to deliver needed fatty acids into the mitochondria. These fatty acids are necessary for keeping brain cells energized, ready for thinking and remembering.

It is thought that carnitine may reverse the loss of brain neurons, impulse-conducting cells. Carnitine also helps prevent the accumulation of intracellular aging pigments while also protecting the brain cell membranes.

Because of its ability to deliver fatty acids to mitochondria, carnitine also has the reputation of helping your heart obtain its peak performance. It has also been shown to improve a damaged heart by allowing the heart to handle stress better.

Others believe carnitine is going to be known for its anti-aging abilities because of its importance in the functioning of mitochondria, which are found in every cell. It may accomplish this by simply keeping the cells healthier by allowing them to obtain all of the fatty acids they need.

Intermittent claudication is a circulatory disease afflicting many people. By allowing fatty deposits to build up in artery walls, intermittent claudication reduces the blood flow to the legs. Less blood also means less oxygen and other nutrients vital to your legs. Beginning symptoms are mild to severe pain in the legs during exertion.

This may develop into more severe symptoms. The skin becomes weak, allowing wounds to occur more easily and heal much more slowly. Pain can develop in the calves, feet, hips, and thighs. In extreme cases, amputation of the affected limb becomes necessary.

Studies done in Italy on the effect carnitine may have on intermittent claudication showed some promising results. One of these studies showed that twelve out of twenty participants had a sixty percent increase in their walking distance. Four participants showed approximately a twenty-five to fifty-nine percent improvement. Four participants showed no improvement in their condition.

Carnitine, added to a daily supplement of coenzyme Q-10, enables you to maintain a healthy lifestyle. For generally healthy people, the recommended dosage is 500 mg daily. Before taking more than this, consult with a knowledgeable health care professional.

CYSTEINE

Cysteine is involved in the creation of taurine, a substance that helps maintain the body's electrical balance. Studies have shown cysteine has the capabilities to reduce the effects of chemotherapy—by reducing chemotherapy's toxicity and lessening the damage to tissues.

Breast milk helps provide cysteine to infants—which is needed for proper development. Cow's milk also contains cysteine, although in lower levels.

GLUTAMINE

Glutamine is a nonessential amino acid that is derived from another nonessential amino acid, glutamic acid. The primary function of glutamine is to act as a detoxifier, especially in the brain.

Glutamine has the capability to cross over the blood–brain barrier, a defense shield surrounding the brain to protect it from toxins. Glutamine helps clear the brain cells of the ammonia that is created during the breakdown process of protein.

Extra ammonia can lead to irritability and even hallucinations. Once inside the brain, glutamine binds with ammonia, then carries it back out of the brain.

Glutamine is considered a necessary part of the healing process by some health care providers for their critically ill surgical patients. Some hospitals routinely use glutamine as a boost to their patients' immunity systems and to hasten recovery.

GLUTAMIC ACID

Glutamic acid is found in plant and animal tissue and is often used as a seasoning to intensify flavors. Glutamic acid is another of the amino acids that has the ability to cross the blood–brain barrier, often transporting potassium.

While in the brain, glutamic acid is used as a fuel. It also detoxifies ammonia found in the brain. Often used to treat personality disorders, glutamic acid has been used in the treatment of childhood behavioral problems, epilepsy, and mental retardation.

Some health care providers check the level of glutamic acid in their patients to detect at an early stage the risk of insulin-dependent diabetes. Glutamic acid is often used to treat a diabetic who has lapsed into a diabetic coma. Researchers are hopeful that in the future glutamic acid will prove beneficial in slowing down the progression of diabetes.

GLYCINE

Although one of glycine's most important roles as a nonessential amino acid is to be an ingredient in making other amino acids, it does have other functions as well. One function is to relieve symptoms of schizophrenia. Symptoms such as emotional unresponsiveness and inexpressiveness are often helped by glycine taken in high doses.

Another brain disorder, hyperactivity, is often treated with glycine. It may also help prevent or lessen the severity of epileptic seizures. Patients suffering from bipolar depression—which used to be called manic depression and is characterized by extreme high moods and low moods—are often helped when taking high doses of glycine.

Alzheimer's disease patients also have reported improvement in brain functions when taking glycine supplements. Improvements in both memory and recall abilities have been observed. These same improvements have been found in healthy adults.

Another health benefit of glycine for the male population is that glycine has been found to improve prostate health.

HISTIDINE

Histidine is a nonessential amino acid released by the immune system that helps with digestion. It accomplishes this task by increasing the secretion of stomach acids. People lacking adequate amounts of stomach acid needed for proper digestion often discover histidine is a helpful source to create additional stomach acid.

Dilating small blood vessels is another duty of histidine. Histidine is also required for the growth and repair of tissues and helps protect the body from radiation damage.

Nerve cells are insulated and protected by myelin sheaths, which also help facilitate the transmission of nerve impulses. Histidine is one of the ingredients needed to maintain these myelin sheaths.

Removing heavy metals from the body is another important role for histidine. Histidine is a necessary component for the production of red and white blood cells. Red blood cells transport oxygen and carbon dioxide back and forth to the tissues. White blood cells help protect the body from infection. Researchers are investigating whether or not this discovery may be helpful in the treatment of AIDS in the future.

High levels of histidine have been found in patients suffering from schizophrenia. Low levels have been discovered in patients suffering from nerve deafness, a hearing disorder, and in patients with rheumatoid arthritis. Another benefit of histidine is that one of its derivatives, histamine, aids those suffering from a lack of sexual arousal.

PROLINE

Proline is a nonessential amino acid that the body produces in lesser amounts than most other amino acids. Proline can be found in most proteins, including those that make up collagen. Collagen is a component of bone, cartilage, skin, tendons, and other connective tissues. Proline also helps to strengthen and heal the cartilage in joints, tendons—even the heart muscle.

Proline can appear to delay the aging process by helping improve skin texture and reducing the loss of collagen in more obvious places, like skin. It also promotes faster wound healing.

Proline levels often become depleted when you are under great stress, you have an infection, you have just undergone surgery, or you have suffered trauma—especially a burn, where wound healing is vital to the healing process.

SERINE

Serine is a nonessential amino acid that is synthesized from another nonessential amino acid—glycine. Serine helps to maintain a healthy immune system, allowing you to fight off infection. It is also needed for the metabolism, or breakdown, of fats that you take in.

Serine is often included as a moisturizer in many skin care products on the market today.

TYROSINE

Tyrosine, a nonessential amino acid, is often associated with depression, other mood disorders, and chronic fatigue syndrome. A higher level of tyrosine helps increase your adrenalin, helping to increase energy and alleviate fatigue. Low levels are associated with hypothyroidism—a disease characterized by reduced energy levels and feeling cold. Tyrosine is used to treat fatigue and anxiety.

Tyrosine helps produce norepinephrine and dopamine, both of which are neurotransmitters necessary to the brain, heart, and central nervous system. It is used to treat Parkinson's disease and to reduce anxiety, including the anxiety and other symptoms suffered when going through drug withdrawal.

Melanin, a pigment responsible for the coloring in skin and hair, is produced by tyrosine. Low blood pressure and low body temperature are two signs of a tyrosine deficiency.

ESSENTIAL FATTY ACIDS

Every body needs some fat. The trick is to take the right kind of fat. Fatty acids are necessary for good health. They also are not manufactured by the body when you need more. They must come in through either diet or supplementation.

Essential fatty acids are found in the highest amounts in the brain and are needed for its normal development and functioning processes. Fatty acids help transmit nerve impulses. Fatty acids are also noted for their ability to:

- ▲ Reduce blood pressure
- ▲ Lower cholesterol and triglyceride levels
- ▲ Reduce the risk of forming blood clots
- ▲ Help to prevent arthritis

A deficiency of fatty acids can lessen your ability to learn and memorize information, and can contribute to higher blood pressure and cholesterol.

There are two types of fatty acids: Omega-3 fatty acids—including eicosapentaenoic acid (**EPA**) and docosahexaenoic acid (**DHA**)—and omega-6 fatty acids—including linoleic acid and gamma-linolenic acids (**GLA**).

Essential fatty acids are widely available in supplement form. Some stores carry a supplement that combines both omega-3 and omega-6 fatty acids. They are also available in foods such as fish oil, salmon, herring, sardines, flax seeds, primrose oil, grape seed oil, and walnut oil.

EICOSAPENTAENOIC ACID (EPA)

Eicosapentaenoic acid is one of the omega-3 essential fatty acids. Studies have shown that it may decrease lung damage in patients with cystic fibrosis. When treated with EPA, cystic fibrosis patients report a decrease in the amount of sputum production and improved lung functions.

EPA has also been linked to the ability to suppress the growth of breast cancer cells and pancreatic cancer cells.

DOCOSAHEXAENOIC ACID (DHA)

Decosahexaenoic acid is another one of the omega-3 essential fatty acids that cannot be produced by the body.

Like EPA, it has been shown to suppress the growth of breast cancer cells. It also has been shown to lower the triglyceride levels, both after fasting and after a meal.

LINOLEIC ACID

Linoleic acid is an essential omega-6 fatty acid especially needed for fetal and infant development and growth. Linoleic acid optimizes the nutritional growth of formula-fed infants by contributing to the efficiency of the formula. It is most often used in infants suffering from cystic fibrosis, which makes absorption of vital nutrients difficult.

Linoleic acid has been shown to reduce the risk of cancers.

GAMMA LINOLENIC ACID (GLA)

Gamma linolenic acid was used by the pilgrims, who were taught of its benefits by the Indians, who used the oil from evening primrose plant seeds as an anti-inflammatory medicine. The pilgrims, duly impressed, sent some back to England, where it became a popular cure-all.

GLA is manufactured by the body from linoleic acid, another essential omega-6 acid. A high-fat diet decreases the production of GLA. Being overweight also reduces production levels. Some people are deficient simply due to heredity.

GLA may prevent heart attacks, breast cancer, diabetes, multiple sclerosis, and rheumatoid arthritis. There are health care providers currently using GLA in the treatment of attention deficit disorder, multiple sclerosis, rheumatoid arthritis, and even schizophrenia. So far, results have been promising.

For infants, breast milk is the best source for GLA. Infants fed breast milk instead of a commercially prepared formula have been shown to have increased immune systems during their breastfeeding days—and up to six months after stopping breast feeding.

One study showed that fifty percent of women suffering from premenstrual symptoms of depression, irritability, breast pain, breast tenderness, and fluid retention reported moderate to complete relief from the symptoms after using GLA.

OTHER SUPPLEMENTS

The number and type of supplements available is always growing. Here are a few other common supplements to consider.

DHEA (DEHYDROEPIANDROSTERONE)

With that long name you can see why it is commonly referred to **DHEA**. DHEA is just one of over 100 hormones produced by the adrenal gland, one of two glands located above each kidney. DHEA's function in your body is to convert itself to estrogen or testosterone on an "as needed" basis. DHEA is currently being touted as a "miracle" supplement. Some claim it:

- ▲ Increases a sense of well-being
- ▲ Slows the aging process
- ▲ Increases production of some types of immune cells
- ▲ May enhance your sex life
- ▲ May help prevent breast cancer
- ▲ May help in the treatment of type II diabetes, cancer, obesity, multiple sclerosis, rheumatoid arthritis, and lupus erythematosus
- ▲ May prevent heart disease

What a list! No wonder some stores can't keep it on the shelves. But many of the claims have yet to be proven. As always, you need to weigh the benefits against any possible risks from taking DHEA.

Possible side effects include:

▲ Acne

▲ Excessive body hair, especially in women

▲ Deepening of a woman's voice

▲ May stimulate the growth of existing prostate or endometrial cancer

Any possible long-term side effects are not currently known.

If you decide to give DHEA a try, start with a small dose and gradually work up to a larger dose. For women, gradual work up to a maximum dose of 25 mg. For men, gradual work up to a maximum dose of 50 mg.

Because DHEA can be used by the body to create sex hormones, women who have not gone through menopause should check with a health care professional before taking DHEA.

Because of the possibility of DHEA affecting prostate cancer, men should make sure to have regular PSA tests, which is a blood test that looks for prostate cancer. Also, always inform your health care provider that you are taking DHEA to avoid any interactions with other medications that you may be taking.

MELATONIN

Melatonin is another hormone found in your body. It is secreted by the pineal gland, which is a small, pea-sized gland located in the brain. Melatonin is currently a popular supplement—its benefits are being touted by many:

▲ Promotes sleep, reduces insomnia

▲ Alleviates jet lag

▲ Kills some cancer cells

▲ May alleviate heart disease, Alzheimer's disease, diabetes, and **SIDS** (sudden infant death syndrome)

▲ Can lengthen and improve the quality of sleep

- ▲ Helps blind people adjust their 24-hour body rhythm
- ▲ Helps people working "swing" shifts adjust to sleeping during the day
- ▲ Slows aging
- ▲ May improve daytime alertness

Melatonin levels in the body are at their greatest when you are in your childhood, peaking when you are in your twenties. After peaking, the melatonin secreted by your brain gradually decreases as you age.

Melatonin secretion is also decreased by your daily lifestyle. Things such as caffeine, alcohol, and prescription medications may decrease your natural melatonin level. Natural melatonin secretion is also reduced by bright light, either natural or artificial.

Your daily melatonin level peaks at around 2 A.M.–3 A.M. This is the reason why a melatonin supplement may be ideal for someone who works a "swing shift" job. Your body just naturally wants to go to sleep at night, not during the daylight hours. If you do try melatonin to help you sleep during the daytime, make sure you take it soon enough, approximately one hour before going to bed, so that you aren't getting sleepy again during your work time hours.

People who are blind or visually-impaired may also find melatonin supplements to be highly beneficial. Daylight helps our bodies naturally know when to sleep and when to wake. But if you can't see light, your body doesn't automatically know when it is time to sleep or time to wake up. It isn't naturally on a twenty-four-hour schedule like we actually live on. So again, taking melatonin one hour before going to bed should help regulate your body clock.

Mobility is a major part of our society today. You can fly anywhere in the world in just hours. The down side to this is jet lag—the modern traveler's curse. Not every traveler is affected by jet lag—some people seem to adjust automatically. But many are afflicted and it may take days to adjust and feel normal again.

Taking melatonin for the symptoms of jet lag is very simple. Just take one melatonin tablet one hour before going to bed—on the schedule of the new time zone. Using melatonin for one or two

Mood Swings—
see Mental Health

Motor Coordination
Prevention of impairment in infants
Iron, page 74

Mouth
Cold sore prevention and healing
Lysine, page 102
Mouth disease prevention
Molybdenum, page 81

Multiple Sclerosis—
see Nervous System

Muscles
Muscle contractions
Potassium, page 84
Muscle relaxant
Magnesium, page 77

Nausea
Nutrient overdose as a cause
Vitamin D, page 55

Nervous System—
see Mental Health for related information
Nerve protection
Lecithin, page 48
Amyotrophic lateral sclerosis (ALS) symptom relief
Threonine, page 106
Bell's palsy recovery
Lysine, page 102
Epilepsy symptom relief
Glutamic acid, page 113
Glycine, page 113
Healthy nervous system maintenance
Calcium, page 65

Phenylalanine, page 106
Vitamin B$_1$ (Thiamin), page 37
Vitamin B$_3$ (Niacin), page 39
Vitamin B$_{12}$, page 42
Vitamin E, page 55
Multiple sclerosis prevention or relief of symptoms
Copper, page 70
DHEA, page 118
Gamma linolenic acid (GLA), page 117
Iron, page 74
Nerve signal transmission
Magnesium, page 77
Neurological disorders prevention
Iron, page 74
Aspartic acid, page 111
Neural tube defect prevention in a developing fetus
Folic acid, page 45
Parkinson's disease symptom relief
Tyrosine, page 115
Vitamin E, page 56

Neural Tube Defects—
see Nervous System

Osteoarthritis—
see Arthritis, Bones

Osteoporosis—see Bones

Pain—also see Headaches and Migraine Headaches for related information
Relief of pain
Aspartic acid, page 111
Phenylalanine, page 106

Parkinson's Disease—see Nervous System

Periodontal Disease—see Gum Disease

Pneumonia—see Lungs

Pregnancy
General nutritional needs
RDAs, page 16
Potential nutrient overdose
Vitamin A/beta-carotene, page 36

Premenstrual Syndrome (PMS)
Symptom relief
Gamma linolenic acid (GLA), page 117
Magnesium, page 76

Prostate
Prostate cancer prevention
Selenium, page 85
Prostate health maintenance
Glycine, page 113

Rheumatoid Arthritis—see Arthritis, Immune System

Senility—see Mental Health

Seniors
Nutritional requirements
RDAs for men, 51+, page 14
RDAs for women, 51+, page 15
Common nutrient deficiencies in older adults
Vitamins, page 30
Vitamin B_6 (Pyridoxine), page 41
Depression and memory loss reduction

Vitamin B_1 (Thiamin), page 37
Immune response strengthening
Vitamin A/beta-carotene, page 34
Vitamin E, page 55
Stomach acid reduction as a cause of nutrient deficiency
Vitamin A/beta-carotene deficiency, page 34

Schizophrenia—see Mental Health

Scurvy
Prevention
Vitamin C, page 50

Skin
Acne control
Selenium, page 86
Aging signs reduction
DHEA, page 118
Melatonin, page 119
Vitamin C, page 50
Cancer prevention
Selenium, page 85
Healing of wounds
Leucine, page 102
Healthy skin maintenance
Vitamin B_6 (Pyridoxine), page 41
Sun damage prevention
Lycopene (vitamin A/beta-carotene), page 35
Para-amino benzoic acid (PABA), page 48

Sleep
Improving Sleep
Melatonin, page 119

Smoking
Cause of nutrient deficiency
　Folic acid, page 45
　Vitamin C, page 51
Increased risk of cancer with smoking and beta-carotene
　Vitamin A/beta-carotene, page 36

Spina Bifida
Prevention of in developing fetus
　Folic acid, page 45

Stress—see Mental Health

Stroke— see Cardiovascular System

Teeth—also see Bones, Gums for related information
Maintenance of strength
　Vitamin D, page 52
　Calcium, page 65

Thyroid
General thyroid health
　Vitamin A/beta-carotene, page 34
Goiter prevention
　Iodine, page 72

Toxins
Antidote to toxins that cause excessive bleeding
　Vitamin K, page 57
Removal of toxins
　Aspartic acid, page 111
　Coenzyme Q-10, page 96
　Glutamine, page 113
　Histidine, page 114
　Magnesium, page 77
　Methionine, page 105
　Selenium, page 86

　Threonine, page 106

Ulcers
Nutrient deficiency as a cause
　Vitamin A/beta-carotene deficiency, page 34

Vascular Problems— see Cardiovascular System

Vision
Cataract prevention
　Vitamin A/beta-carotene, page 34
　Vitamin B_2 (Riboflavin), page 38
　Vitamin C, page 50
　Vitamin E, page 56
Eye fatigue
　Vitamin B_2 (Riboflavin), page 38
General eye health
　B vitamins, page 36
　Zinc, page 89
Glaucoma control
　Vitamin C, page 50
Macular degeneration prevention
　Vitamin C, page 50

Weight Loss
Nutrient overdose as cause of weight loss
　Vitamin D, page 55

Women—also see Breasts, Pregnancy for related information
Nutritional requirements
　RDAs, page 15

Wound Healing— see Blood, Skin

References

Hundreds of sources were referred to while writing this book. For a list of the references please send a request to:

>   The Crossing Press
>   97 Hangar Way
>   Watsonville, CA 95076
>   831.722.0711

Index

A
acetaminophen overdose, 105
acidic foods, 34
Adequate Intake (AI), 17
adverse affects
   of DHEA, 119
   of excess boron, 64
   of excess folic acid, 48
   of excess molybdenum, 81
   of excess potassium, 85
   of excess sodium, 89
   of excess vitamin B3 (niacin), 40
   of excess vitamin B6 (pyridoxine), 42
   of excess vitamin B12, 44
   of excess vitamin C, 52
   of excess vitamin D, 54-55
   of excess vitamin E, 57
   of excess zinc, 91
   of melatonin, 121
   reporting, 28
   See also nutritional supplements
age
   beta-carotene deficiency and, 34
   as nutritional supplement factor, 20, 93
   optimal amounts of minerals and, 63
alanine, 108-109
alcohol usage
   absorption of B12 and, 44
   alanine levels and, 108-109
   calcium absorption and, 66
   folic acid deficiency and, 45
   melatonin secretion and, 120
   mineral deficiencies and, 62
   nutritional deficits due to, 21
   supplements in case of, 93
allergies, 122
alpha-tocopherol (vitamin E), 30, 31, 32, 55-57
Alzheimer's Disease, 97, 114, 119
American College of Obstetrics and Gynecology, 36
amino acids
   described, 99
   essential, 100-108
   nonessential, 108-116
amyotrophic lateral sclerosis (ALS), 107
anemia, 45
antioxidant labels, 25

antioxidants, 31-32
arginine, 109-110
aspartic acid, 111
attention deficit disorder, 118
AZT, 101

B
beta-carotene, 32, 33-36
biotin, 44
boron, 64
breast cancer, 73
breastfeeding women
    calcium RDAs for, 66
    folic acid RDAs for, 46
    iodine RDAs for, 73
    iron RDAs for, 75
    magnesium RDAs for, 78
    nutritional supplements for, 20
    phosphorus RDAs for, 82
    RDAs for, 16
    selenium RDAs for, 86
    vitamin A/beta-carotene RDAs for, 35
    vitamin B1 (thiamin) RDAs for, 37
    vitamin B2/riboflavin RDAs for, 39
    vitamin B3/niacin RDAs for, 40
    vitamin B6/pyridoxine RDAs for, 42
    vitamin B12 RDAs for, 43
    vitamin C RDAs for, 51
    vitamin D RDAs for, 53
    vitamin E RDAs for, 56
    vitamin K RDAs for, 58
    zinc RDAs for, 90

See also pregnant women;women

C
calcium, 65-68
calcium carbonate, 67
calcium citrate, 67
calcium gluconate, 67
calcium lactate, 67
calcium phosphate, 67
calcium supplements, 55
cancer. *See* nutrients/health condition cross reference
carbohydrates, 8
carnitine, 105, 111-112
catalysts, 29
children
    calcium RDAs for, 66
    copper deficiency in, 70
    folic acid RDAs for, 46
    iodine deficiency in, 73
    iodine RDAs for, 73
    iron deficiency in, 74
    iron RDAs for, 75
    magnesium RDAs for, 78
    phosphorus RDAs for, 82
    RDAs for, 13
    selenium RDAs for, 86
    vitamin A RDAs for, 35
    vitamin B1 (thiamin) RDAs for, 37
    vitamin B2/riboflavin RDAs for, 38
    vitamin B3/niacin RDAs for, 39
    vitamin B6/pyridoxine RDAs for, 42
    vitamin B12 RDAs for, 43

vitamin C RDAs for, 51
vitamin D RDAs for, 53
vitamin E RDAs for, 56
vitamin K RDAs for, 58
zinc RDAs for, 90
See also infants
cholesterol levels, 49, 55
chromium, 68-69
coenzyme Q-10, 96-98, 112
coffee, 66
copper, 69-71
Coumadin, 57
cysteine, 112

D

D-aspartate, 111
Daily Value (DV), 11
depression. *See* nutrients/health condition cross reference
DHEA (dehydroepiandrosterone), 118-119
dietary guidelines, 9-10
Dietary Reference Intakes (DRIs), 17-18
digestive enzymes, 98
diseases. *See* nutrients/health condition cross reference
diuretics, 84
docosahexaenoic acid (DHA), 116, 117
drinkers. *See* alcohol usage

E

eicosapentaenoic acid (EPA), 116, 117
enzymes, 96-98
eosinophilia-myalgia syndrome (EMS), 94
essential amino acids, 100-108
essential fatty acids, 116-118
Estimated Average Requirement (EAR), 17

F

fat, 8
fat-soluble vitamins, 30
FDA MedWatch hotline, 94
Federal Trade Commission (FTC), 24
fertility, 89
fluoride, 71-72
folic acid (folate or folicin), 44-48
Food and Drug Administration (FDA), 24, 25, 28, 93-94, 107
Food Guide Pyramid, 9-10
foods
  beta-carotene absorption and acidic, 34
  boron sources in, 64
  calcium sources in, 65-66
  chromium sources in, 69
  copper sources in, 70-71
  essential fatty acids in, 116
  folic acid sources in, 47
  iodine sources in, 73
  iron sources in, 75-76
  lysine sources in, 104
  macronutrients in, 7-9
  magnesium sources in, 78
  manganese sources in, 80
  methionine sources in, 105
  mineral deficiencies of overcooked, 62

molybdenum sources in, 81
phosphorus sources in, 83
potassium sources in, 84
selenium sources in, 87
threonine sources in, 107
tryptophan sources in, 107
vitamin A/beta-carotene sources in, 35
vitamin B12 sources in, 43
vitamin C sources in, 51-52
vitamin D sources in, 54
vitamin E sources in, 56
vitamin K sources in, 59
zinc sources in, 91
free radicals, 31-32, 102

G
gamma-linolenic acids (GLA), 116, 117-118
genital herpes, 103
glutamic acid, 113
glutamine, 113
glycine, 113-114
granola product nutrition facts, 11

H
HDL cholesterol levels, 49
health condition/nutrients cross reference, 123-133
hepatitis, 108, 122
herpes, 103-104, 110, 122
high potency labels, 25
histidine, 114-115
hyperactivity, 114
hypothyroidism, 115

I
IAZT, 101
impotence, 109
incontinence, 105
infants
    calcium RDAs for, 66
    folic acid RDAs for, 46
    iodine RDAs for, 73
    iron RDAs for, 75
    magnesium RDAs for, 78
    needs for alanine by, 109
    phosphorus RDAs for, 82
    RDAs for, 13
    selenium RDAs for, 86
    SIDS (sudden infant death syndrome) in, 119
    vitamin A RDAs for, 35
    vitamin B1/thiamin RDAs for, 37
    vitamin B2/riboflavin RDAs for, 38
    vitamin B3/niacin RDAs for, 39
    vitamin B6/pyridoxine RDAs for, 42
    vitamin B12 RDAs for, 43
    vitamin C RDAs for, 51
    vitamin D RDAs for, 53
    vitamin E RDAs for, 56
    vitamin K RDAs for, 58
    zinc RDAs for, 90
    See also children
insomnia, 107, 119
intermittent claudication, 112
iodine, 72-74
iron, 74-76
iron deficiency, 74-75
iron supplements, 76

isoleucine, 101-102
IU (international unit), 18

L
L-trytophan, 94
laxatives, 84
LDL cholesterol levels, 49, 55
lecithin (phosphatidylcholine or PC), 48
leucine, 102
linoleic acid, 116, 117
Lou Gehrig's disease, 97
lupus erythematosus, 118, 122
lutein, 34-35
lycopene, 34-35
lysine, 102-104

M
macronutrients, 7-9
magnesium, 76-79
magnesium deficiency, 77
magnesium supplements, 79
manganese, 79-80
Maple Syrup Urine Disease (MSUD), 101
mcg (microgram), 18
melatonin, 119-121
men
　calcium RDAs for, 66
　folic acid RDAs for, 46
　impotence in, 109
　infertility in, 50, 79, 89
　iodine RDAs for, 73
　iron RDAs for, 75
　magnesium RDAs for, 78
　phosphorus RDAs for, 82
　RDAs for, 14
　selenium RDAs for, 86
　vitamin B1 (thiamin) RDAs for, 37
　vitamin B2/riboflavin RDAs for, 38
　vitamin B3/niacin RDAs for, 39-40
　vitamin B6/pyridoxine RDAs for, 42
　vitamin B12 RDAs for, 43
　vitamin C RDAs for, 51
　vitamin D RDAs for, 53
　vitamin E RDAs for, 56
　vitamin K RDAs for, 58
　zinc RDAs for, 90
Meniere's disease, 104
methionine, 105
mg (milligram), 18
mineral deficiencies, 62-63
mineral supplements, 63
mineral toxicity, 63
minerals
　boron, 64
　calcium, 65-68
　chromium, 68-69
　copper, 69-71
　described, 8, 60
　fluoride, 71-72
　functions of, 60-61
　macromineral/microminerals listed, 61-62
mitochondria, 111-112
molybdenum, 80-81
multivitamin/multimineral supplement, 12
　See also nutritional supplements

INDEX ▲ 139

N

N-methyl, 111
National Academy of Science (NAS), 11
National Institute of Medicine (NIM), 11, 33
niacin or nicotinic acid (vitamin B3), 39-40
NMDA, 111
nonessential amino acids, 108-116
nutrients/health condition cross reference, 123-133
nutrition
    components of food, 7-9
    facts on granolo product, 11
nutritional supplements
    amino acids, 99-116
    avoiding excessive use of, 27-28
    boron, 64
    calcium, 66-68
    categories of, 95
    chromium, 69
    combinations of, 27
    common forms of, 94-95
    copper in multivitamin/multimineral, 71
    during stress/exposure to toxins, 21
    enzymes, 96-98
    essential fatty acids, 116-118
    facts on multivitamin/multimineral, 12
    folic acid, 47
    getting advice on, 25-26
    inability to eat normal diet and, 21
    increasing age and, 20
    iron, 76
    knowing source of, 26-27
    magnesium, 79
    need for nonherbal, 92-93
    perspective on, 5-6
    phosphorus, 83
    safety of, 93-94
    special circumstances for, 20-21
    to enhance health/well-being, 23
    to prevent certain health problems, 22
    to treat certain health conditions, 21-22
    understanding risks of, 24-25
    vitamin B12, 44
    vitamin D, 54
    vitamin E, 57
    vitamin K, 59
    wise purchase of, 27
    zinc, 91
    See also adverse affects;Recommended Dietary Allowances (RDA)

O

omega-3 fatty acids, 116, 117
omega-6 fatty acids, 116, 117
oral contraceptives, 45
osteoporosis, 64

P

pain. *See* nutrients/health condition cross reference
pangamic acid (vitamin B15), 44
pantothenic acid (vitamin B5), 41
para-amino benzoic acid (PABA), 48
Pauling, Linus, 48
phenylalanine, 106
phosphatidylcholine or PC, 48
phosphorus, 82-83
potassium, 83-85
pregnant women
   calcium RDAs for, 66
   folic acid RDAs for, 46
   iodine RDAs for, 73
   iron RDAs for, 75
   magnesium RDAs for, 78
   nutritional supplements for, 20
   phosphorus RDAs for, 82
   RDAs for, 16
   selenium RDAs for, 86
   vitamin A/beta-carotene RDAs for, 35, 36
   vitamin B1 (thiamin) RDAs for, 37
   vitamin B2/riboflavin RDAs for, 39
   vitamin B3/niacin RDAs for, 40
   vitamin B6/pyridoxine RDAs for, 42
   vitamin B12 RDAs for, 43
   vitamin C RDAs for, 51
   vitamin D RDAs for, 53
   vitamin E RDAs for, 56
   vitamin K RDAs for, 58
   zinc RDAs for, 90
   See also breastfeeding women;women
proline, 115
proteins, 8
psoriasis, 122
pyridoxine (vitamin B6), 41-42

R

RDI (Reference Daily Intake), 12
Recommended Dietary Allowances (RDA)
   antioxidants, 32
   boron, 64
   calcium, 66
   described, 11-12
   as DRI category, 17
   folate, 46
   for infants/children, 13
   iodine, 73
   iron, 75
   magnesium, 78
   manganese, 79
   for men, 14
   note about vitamin, 33
   phosphorus, 82
   for pregnant/breastfeeding women, 16
   selenium, 86
   sodium, 88
   on supplement labels, 27
   used as baseline, 18
   vitamin A (beta-carotene), 35
   vitamin B1 (thiamin), 37

vitamin B2, 38-39
vitamin B2 (riboflavin), 38-39
vitamin B3 (niacin), 39-40
vitamin B6 (pyridoxine), 42
vitamin B12, 43
vitamin C, 51
vitamin D, 53
vitamin E (alpha-tocopherol), 56
vitamin K, 58
for women, 15
zinc, 90
See also nutritional supplements
riboflavin (vitamin B2), 38-39

S

selenium, 85-87
serine, 115
sexually transmitted diseases (STDs), 122
SIDS (sudden infant death syndrome), 119
sinus problems, 122
smoking. *See* nutrients/health condition cross reference
sodium, 87-89
stress. *See* nutrients/health condition cross reference
supplement labels
  FDA guidelines on, 24-25
  RDAs on, 27
  See also nutritional supplements

T

T-cells, 106, 110
thiamin (vitamin B1), 36-37
threonine, 106-107
thymic factors, 122
Tolerable Upper Intake Level (TUIL), 17
toxin exposure, 21
tryptophan, 107
tyrosine, 106, 115-116

U

ultraviolet (UV) rays, 53

V

valine, 108
vitamin A, 30, 33-36
vitamin B1 (thiamin), 36-37
vitamin B2 (riboflavin), 38-39
vitamin B3 (niacin or nicotinic acid), 39-40
vitamin B5 (pantothenic acid), 41
vitamin B6 (pyridoxine), 41-42
vitamin B12, 30-31, 42-44
vitamin B15 (pangamic acid), 44
vitamin C, 30, 32, 48-52, 123
vitamin D, 30, 52-55
vitamin E (alpha-tocopherol), 30, 31, 32, 55-57
vitamin K, 57-59
vitamin Q (coenzyme Q-10), 96-98, 112
vitamins
  antioxidants, 31-32

described, 8
fat/water-soluble, 30-31
functions of, 29-30
RDAs for, 33

W

warfarin (Coumadin), 57
water-soluble vitamins, 30
women
  calcium RDAs for, 66
  folic acid RDAs for, 46
  iodine RDAs for, 73
  iron RDAs for, 75
  magnesium RDAs for, 78
  phosphorus RDAs for, 82
  RDAs for, 15, 16
  selenium RDAs for, 86
  vitamin A RDAs for, 35
  vitamin B1 (thiamin) RDAs for, 37
  vitamin B2/riboflavin RDAs for, 38
  vitamin B3/niacin RDAs for, 40
  vitamin B6/pyridoxine RDAs for, 42
  vitamin B12 RDAs for, 43
  vitamin C RDAs for, 51
  vitamin D RDAs for, 53
  vitamin E RDAs for, 56
  vitamin K RDAs for, 58
  zinc RDAs for, 90
  See also breastfeeding women;pregnant women
World Health Organization (WHO), 19

Z

zinc, 89-91
zinc deficiency, 90

Other books in the Vital Information Series

Surgery
By Molly Shapiro, M.B.A., R.N.

So, you may be facing surgery. Whether this is your first surgery or not, health care is different today. Surgery covers every aspect of the surgery process including what your rights are as a patient. It tells you how to prepare for surgery, what happens in surgery, explains equipment use and procedures, and answers your post-op concerns.

$11.95 • ISBN 0-89594-898-2

Hospitals
By Diane Barnet, M.S., R.N.

Hospitals can be intimidating places. Many consumers don't know how to obtain information or even what questions to ask. *Hospitals* provides inside information for patients and their advocates. It explains how hospitals function, and includes an overview of our body systems and a user-friendly guide to medical equipment, procedures, and drugs.

$11.95 • ISBN 0-89594-908-3

Perimenopause
By Bernard Cortese, M.D.

Perimenopause describes the changes that may take place during the transitional time before and after menopause, discusses the pros and cons of hormone replacement therapy (HRT), offers alternative treatments, and stresses the importance of exercise, proper diet, and stress management. It is a practical guide that will help all women be better prepared for this stage of life.

$11.95 • ISBN 0-89594-914-8

To receive a current catalog from The Crossing Press,
please call toll-free,
800-777-1048.
Visit our Website on the Internet at: www.crossingpress.com